COPING WITH CANCER

HANDS-ON STRATEGIES FOR MANAGING THE BIG 'C'

RAMENDRA KUMAR

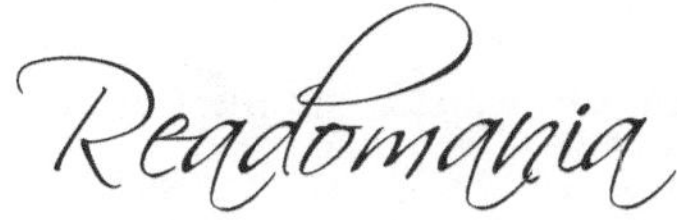

Readomania

An imprint of Kurious Kind Media Private Limited
readomania.com
email: contact@readomania.com
Facebook: facebook.com/iamreadomania
Twitter: twitter.com/iamreadomania
Instagram: iamreadomania

First Published in 2024 by Readomania

Edited by Indrani Ganguly (Managing Editor, Readomania)

ISBN: 978-93-91800-80-2

Typeset in Palatino Linotype by Shine Graphics
Printed in Delhi

*To, my MAA (Madhavi, Ankita & Aniket) for reclaiming
me from the kingdom of the dead three times!*

*My gratitude to my friends for being there throughout
my tortuous cancer journey!*

Contents

Foreword

When Siddhartha Mukherjee, an India born American oncologist, began writing the biography of cancer, and named it *Emperor of All Maladies* (published in 2010), it was not for nothing that he named cancer as an all-pervasive unwinnable scourge of mankind that had remained enigmatic, unconquered, with a potential to destroy a person afflicted by it. Even in the 19th century, cancer was described as the 'king of terror'.

Though, in the last five decades, medical science has made significant advancement in the understanding of cancer, in terms of aetiology, genetics, its management by various modalities, prognosis, and outcome; yet, cancer has defied all logic and reason, and keeps on baffling patients and doctors alike. However, in the last two or three decades, real advancement has been made on how people afflicted by cancer have used various coping mechanisms and styles to improve on the outcome of the illness.

In this book, *Coping With Cancer*: *Hands-on strategies for managing the Big 'C'*, Ramendra Kumar has added remarkable understanding on what a person or family could do when faced with an uncertain future as a result of cancer diagnosis. In a bold measure, he has narrated his own experiences with cancer, and how his family provided all the support in going through this journey. He has also described how some celebrities battled this illness at the prime of their career.

Through his own journey and of others, Ramendra has identified eleven coping strategies. Under each mechanism he has detailed the experience of a patient or caregiver, and how others in similar situations can employ these concepts.

The entire narration is in simple and lucid language, and makes a lasting impression on the reader. Though of late, a number of books have appeared in the market authored by a cancer survivor (or, one may say, cancer warrior), where the author describes his or her own journey with the disease, this book is remarkably different. It is a 'self-help' guide that fills a long-felt gap in this space. All the stakeholders, namely, patients, families, doctors, counsellors and NGOs working in this field will find it immensely useful.

PROF. SUDHIR K. KHANDELWAL, MD, MRC, PSYCHIATRY
Senior Consultant in Psychiatry
Holy Family Hospital, New Delhi
Former, Head, Dept. of Psychiatry and
Chief, National Drug Dependence Treatment Centre
All India Institute of Medical Sciences

Preface

Fighting Every Tumour with Humour!

Just as the pure white lotus flower blooms unsoiled in muddy water, our lives, which are supremely noble, can continue to shine even amid life's harshest realities.

—Daisaku Ikeda,
Japanese Buddhist philosopher & author

My wife Madhavi and I took Voluntary Retirement in August 2020, from SAIL, Rourkela Steel Plant, where we were serving as General Managers. We shifted to Bengaluru where our children Ankita and Aniket are working.

This period was the best in my life. I wrote two books, one of which topped the charts on Amazon in its category. I was invited to literary fests, webinars, storytelling sessions and workshops and the response was humongous.

In early November, I was suffering from slight, or what I thought were slight, issues of indigestion. I went to the gastroenterologist. He prescribed some medicines and asked me to report back to him after two weeks. A day before I was to consult him, I saw two teaspoons of blood in my stool. We rushed to the doctor and he suggested a colonoscopy which was carried out. Subsequently, a biopsy was also done.

On 29th November at around noon, I was sitting with Madhavi and our children in the doctor's chamber. He went through the reports, had a look at a few slides and delivered his verdict in a matter-of-fact way, as if he was reading the weather report on Doordarshan.

"The reports have come and I have looked at them. Mr. Kumar, you have colorectal cancer."

Even as my brain was processing this information, I heard him say, "Your colon is infested with multiple polyps which are hanging like grapes. One of the polyps is already cancerous and a couple more are in the pre-cancerous stage."

"H…how long do I have?" I managed to ask, feeling a huge sense of déjà vu. Though I had heard this question in countless movies, never in my wildest imagination had I ever thought I would be sitting in front of a doctor popping this query at him.

The Gastroenterologist looked at me impassively. "Mr. Kumar, if ever one must choose any cancer—then colorectal cancer is the best bet. Besides, fortunately your cancer is only between the 2nd and 3rd stages. I would advise that you start the treatment immediately."

"What will it entail?" Madhavi asked.

"We will have to carry out some blood tests and scans. This will be followed by a short aggressive treatment of five rounds of daily targeted radiation and four to five cycles of chemo. After which he will have to undergo a major surgery wherein his colon will be totally removed and the small intestine brought out. He will be fitted with a stoma bag to collect the stool for a minimum of three weeks. Depending on how his body responds, the surgery for reconnecting the small intestine to the rectum would be performed and the stoma bag will, hopefully, be done away with. Thereafter, he will have to undergo another five cycles of chemo."

We went and sat in the canteen. I was in a complete daze.

"How the hell could God do this to me? I don't smoke, I don't drink, I am not overweight, I exercise regularly, I don't take much of red meat—then how come me?" I went through the entire spectrum of anger, agony, angst, frustration and yes, even a few tears.

I looked at Madhavi, Anki and Ani. Their faces seemed to simply crumple. It was as if they were seeing my death in my own eyes.

It was then, at that very moment, I decided I couldn't subject my family to the trauma I was going through! After all, I have always believed that family comes first.

Throughout my life I had battled the toughest of odds in my own way. I was a suicide survivor and the product of a broken home when I was 15.

Even my marriage to Madhavi had been a tough one involving lots of struggle and sacrifice on both our parts. Ours was an inter-caste marriage and her parents were dead against it. As a result, I had to resign from my job and rejoin later. I was junior to Madhavi and my batchmates for more than a decade and faced a lot of ridicule and shame. She too was estranged from her family for three years. Finally, her parents reconciled and I too made up the shortfall.

Susan Sontag, in her seminal book *Illness as Metaphor*, writes, "Everyone who is born holds dual citizenship—in the kingdom of the well and in the kingdom of the sick. Although we all prefer to use only the good passport, sooner or later each of us is obliged, at least for a spell, to identify ourselves as citizens of that other place."

However, in my life my passport to the 'kingdom of the sick' had been stamped not once or twice but on several occasions. I am a patient of brittle diabetes where the sugar levels oscillate from the extreme low to the extreme high within 12 hours. To manage this condition, I have been fitted permanently with an insulin pump. I also suffer from silent thyroiditis in which too the swings are extreme. In 2011, I had a tryst with TB. A few years later I was diagnosed with a rare condition in which there was a polyp growing close to my vocal cords and there was a danger of me losing my voice. I was rushed to Hyderabad where a critical surgery was performed and normalcy was restored.

I had battled all these 'scourges' with my exclusive mantra of 'Managing every tumour with humour'. And now when I was facing the biggest challenge of my life, positivity was the only choice.

Being a writer, a storyteller and an inspirational speaker, my response had to be different. I had to forge a new reality, script my own story, live it and love it.

I decided to wage a war against cancer with my credo, my mantra.

I am a cancer warrior having endured 3 septic shocks (the probability of surviving one septic shock is only around 30%), 4 major surgeries, 5 rounds of radiation, 10 chemo cycles and 40 days in the ICU.

After a gruelling battle with the Big 'C' which lasted close to a year, I was finally declared cancer free in November 2022.

During the entire journey, from the diagnosis, to the pre-surgery treatment, to the post-surgery recovery, I tried my best to remain upbeat. I participated in panel discussions, interviews, posted poems and parodies. I filled social media with messages of hope and optimism—I was certainly down, but by no means out!

My greatest support system throughout this terrible ordeal has been my family. The lives of my seraphs had become a relentless syndrome of visits to the hospital, meetings with the doctors, a few hours at home and back again—each moment alternating between dread and relief, despair and hope. But in all this chaos none of them pressed the panic button. And whenever I had my brief rendezvous with them, they never, ever gave me a glimpse of the Hades in which I was existing.

My foul weather friends unleashed a fusillade of love, concern and blessings. Lamps were lit and offerings made in several temples, *duas* were recited in masjids from Lahore to Lucknow to Guwahati, special prayers were organised in churches, in gurudwaras, friends sent me Buddhist chants, Vedic mantras and healing invocations. Columns in newspapers, and posts on social media lauded my resilience. A writer buddy of mine compared me to Raphael Nadal who played Wimbledon even while battling a serious injury! Another friend said I was Anand 2.0. I was called a messiah, an inspiration, even given the sobriquet Ramen SherKhan! The Indian Cancer Society invited me for their online and offline sessions, my experience on my fight with the malady was published in national and international platforms and I was called to literary festivals to share my cancer journey. My onco surgeon made a documentary on my positivity. Madhavi and my love story in the backdrop of cancer was showcased by 'Humans of Bombay', one of the most popular pages on Instagram. The reel went viral notching up more than 4 million views.

I was simply amazed at the love, affection, concern and blessings I was inundated with. My family, my friends and I managed to create an ecosystem of positivity—a universe, which helped me claw back, quite literally, from the jaws of death.

I now carry a stoma bag with me to collect the waste matter. This means a significant adjustment in my lifestyle and restrictions on my movement. The doctors are of the opinion that any surgery to remove the stoma bag and restore the status quo might prove fatal. Hence the bag too, like the insulin pump, is my forever companion.

Besides, every night as I lie down there are several other harsh reminders of my condition. I suffer a terrible pain in my toes, shin and calf muscles. The bottoms of my feet feel like they are being pierced by innumerable needles! This goes on for close to thirty minutes, after which I slowly drift into sleep.

When I consulted my doctor he said, "Mr. Kumar, we have no precedence for what you have gone through. You probably know by now that we had given up on you three times! Therefore, we do not want to prescribe any more drugs. If the pain is not intolerable, please bear with it. It is a neuropathic issue and should hopefully resolve over a period of time."

I have often been asked why I am so open about my journey.

My response is simple: "As a family we have always believed in truth and transparency. Ever since the diagnosis slammed into me, I have made an effort to be candid about the challenges I was facing. My logic is that when I have shared the 'best of times' with my friends, why shouldn't I share the 'worst of times'? Besides, there is nothing to be ashamed of—I am not responsible for my cancer—I have done nothing to deserve it. The reason is genetic (my mother apparently had colorectal cancer but it was misdiagnosed as piles) and there is nothing I can do about it—except to fight the illness.

Also, I felt if by reaching out I could make even a slightest of difference for the better, in the lives of others, my effort would be more than worth it. My approach has been validated with quite a few of the patients and their caregivers connecting with me and sharing their journey and seeking advice.

This book, I hope, will be my most significant contribution and prove to be a hands-on compendium for anyone who is coping with cancer.

RAMENDRA KUMAR
Bengaluru, 2024

Coping Strategies

1. Learning to accept

2. Living in the present moment

3. Normalising

4. Creating an ecosystem of positivity

5. Connecting with self

6. Investing in relationships

7. Finding a sense of purpose

8. Building resilience

9. Pursuing a passion

10. Moving from fear to faith

11. Taking humour seriously

1

Learning to Accept

Acceptance doesn't mean resignation; it means understanding that something is what it is and that there's got to be a way through it.

—MICHAEL J. FOX, *Canadian-American actor*

In almost all cases when the cancer verdict slams into the patient or his/her caregiver, the first reaction is denial. This sentiment is invariably followed by confusion, anger, frustration and the tendency to blame God, karma *et al*.

In this situation one can draw inspiration from The Serenity Prayer, which guides the Alcoholic Anonymous movement: *God, grant me the serenity to accept the things I cannot change, the courage to change the things I can, and the wisdom to know the difference.*

In his book *Introspective Meditations for Complete Contentment (Santosha)*, Manoj Sharma, writes, "Acceptance starts with us. We must accept the body and mind the way we are. Acceptance has to be inculcated at the thought, words and action level..."

The earlier the afflicted and the affected learn to accept the diagnosis and move forward the more effective and impacting is the result.

Lachlan Brown, the author of *Hidden Secrets of Buddhism* says he has learned that acceptance is the cornerstone of inner peace. When we accept that nothing and no one, including ourselves, is perfect, we begin to let go. We stop caring about the non-essential things. He emphasises on the Zen concept of *wabi-sabi* which teaches the art of finding beauty in imperfection and is essentially about appreciating things as they are, not how you think they should be.

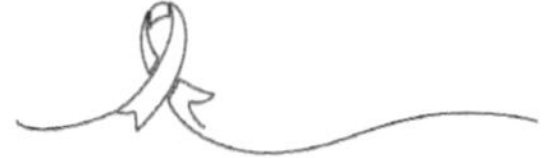

Case Study I: Mukta Sharma[1]

When Mukta's six-year-old niece, Riya (name changed) was diagnosed with blood cancer, the entire family was devastated. To think that such a young child could have a life-threatening disease seemed something impossible to cope with. However, soon every one rallied around to do everything they could for the youngest member of the close-knit family.

Mukta took the first flight to be by Riya's side through the entire course of treatment. Keeping a little girl engaged through the long and arduous days of chemotherapy was not easy. Mukta took up the task using all her ingenuity. She thought up of little games, mimed dialogues from the TV serials they watched and created moments of fun in the simplest of ways.

Since Riya was missing school and also the company of her grandparents and elder sister, the biggest challenge for Mukta was to ensure that the little angel's spirits were kept high. To do this she herself had to be upbeat. Mukta would

---

[1] To protect the privacy of patients and caregivers, names have been changed. When only the first names are used, they are fictitious. However, when full names are given, these are actual names.

recite the Gayatri Mantra, sing Jagjit Singh's songs out loud and do whatever else that helped soothe her often frayed nerves and keep her in a positive state of mind.

What is her advice to cancer caregivers? Accept the situation. You cannot change it by being angry or sad. Cancer cannot be wished away. Having a cheerful attitude can make the entire experience easier for you and for the patient.

Giving her own example, Mukta says she has always been a moody person. If she was upset, it took days for her to cheer up again. She was protected by her family all her life, and never had to cope with problems. She feels that if someone like her can be a cancer caregiver, then anyone can. Cancer has a way of teaching you how to manage the ups and downs.

While she still chokes up when she recalls those days of turbulence, Mukta feels that it's important to remain optimistic and look for simple things to motivate you through your journey as a caregiver.

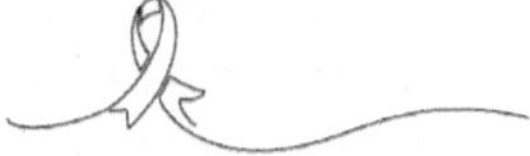

Case Study II: Sudha

Sudha was diagnosed with second stage breast cancer. Just three months ago she had lost her husband Pavan to the same dreaded disease. The family had traversed the tortuous and torturous journey for years with the hope that he would pull through. Sudha's *Amma*, Usha (name changed) and she had tried everything—the best doctors, a reputed hospital, they had spent all their energy and effort and had bled their finances but to no avail. And now, just as she was recovering from the shock of his death, she had been struck by the same deadly sickness!

Sudha writes about her immediate reaction on coming to know about her cancer.

"As the black wave of depression hit me, I stumbled out of the hospital. I felt myself sinking into a never-ending abyss, my mind completely blank. I somehow managed to get an auto rickshaw and reach home. I was a bit relieved that no one would be there. Amma had taken my son Sudhir to the therapist. I needed time before I could face her or anyone else.

I let myself in with the spare key and collapsed on the bed. In just an hour my world had once again crumbled. The doctor's verdict had been terse, 'Mrs. Sudha, you have breast cancer, 2nd stage and we need to start the treatment as early as possible...'

After that I couldn't recollect anything except disconnected words....Radiation...chemo...surgery...it was all a blur."

Lying in bed, she began to curse her fate. How could God be so cruel to her? Within a few months of seeing her husband succumb to cancer she had fallen prey to the same deadly malaise. A black wave of depression hit her.

More than feel a sense of self pity, Sudha was swamped by her concern for Usha. How much more would she have to endure in just one lifetime? She had lost her husband when she was just 38. She was left with a meagre income of a clerk in a bank and the humongous responsibility of bringing up three children. She had fought through it all with a resilience which was truly rare. Adversity had always been a constant companion. Even while the family was battling Pavan's illness there was another shocker. Her grandson was diagnosed with clinical depression and she with gall bladder stones. *Amma* had taken everything in her stride, battling each skirmish with grit and gumption. But now, at the age of 73, did she deserve this brutal blow?

Sudha goes on to narrate *Amma's* reaction to the diagnosis and the indelible impact it left on her.

"As soon as *Amma* entered the house with Sudhir in tow she asked, 'What did the doctor say?'

'Nothing much, just some infection,' I told her, even as I avoided meeting her eyes.

After Sudhir had gone to his room, she turned towards me. 'Sudha, I know you are trying to hide something. Tell me, what is the finding?'

I told her and as *Amma* held me, the tears just wouldn't stop.

She let me cry and then making me sit on the bed began talking to me, 'There is always a meaning behind every problem that we face in our life. I am sure the Almighty has thrown this challenge with a purpose. Let us accept it with grace and fight with courage.'

And with these words *Amma* simply took charge of everything."

Usha accompanied her daughter to almost every visit to the hospital as well as went along with her grandson on his trips to the therapist. She cooked all the meals making sure Sudha had only the prescribed diet. She managed the finances adroitly, dipping into her meagre savings whenever necessity arose.

Sudha was frequently afflicted by doubts whether all the money, time, energy and effort *Amma* was devoting to her treatment were really worth it. What was the guarantee that like Pawan, Sudha too would not succumb to cancer?

Whenever Sudha would share her qualms *Amma* would respond with earthy wisdom.

"Sudha, all of us have to die one day and cancer is not the one and only reason that people expire. Just because Pavan succumbed to the illness does not mean that you too will not survive. Let us give our best and pray for the rest."

Throughout Sudha's cancer journey, her mother never once expressed doubts about everything not going as expected. She filled the atmosphere with positivity which was crucial. Her attitude reinforced her daughter's belief in the effectiveness of the treatment. Her optimism became Sudha's greatest weapon in her battle with cancer.

Finally, more than a year after her diagnosis, Sudha was declared cancer free.

Sudha offers a heartfelt tribute to her mother.

"*Amma* was a pillar of strength in dealing with the various issues that I faced during the period. Like it is generally done, *Amma* never blamed my destiny or the Almighty. She never clinically dissected nor critically analysed. She simply offered her unconditional acceptance to every situation.

The reason I am emphasising my mother's huge contribution in helping me cope with my disease is to reiterate to caregivers the importance of their support and positive response for the cancer patient. Morale of the patient keeps undulating depending upon the severity of physical stress and strain. She is uncertain about the efficacy of cure as well as her lifespan. The patient tends to form an opinion about the success of treatment depending upon the atmosphere around her. In such a scenario the frame of mind and attitude of caregivers makes a crucial difference.

Amma swallowed all the hardships like a sea which swallows water from all the rivers that flow into it. By looking at the beautiful white waves we can never imagine how much water, dirt and waste have entered the sea. Just like the sea, *Amma* too stood by me, accepting the entire physical, mental and emotional trauma and providing support and consolation."

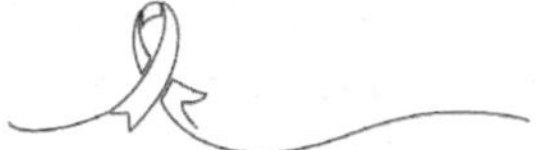

Case Study III: Pallavi Aiyar

Pallavi is a journalist and author, who was diagnosed with breast cancer in August 2022. She lost her mother Gitanjali Aiyar, the well-known Doordarshan newsreader, in June 2023.

Her response is a classic case of how the diagnosis and the aftermath can be dealt with.

"Cancer is not an illness as much as a metaphor for life's deadly fragility. The weight of the word in the mouth, conjures up bald heads and painful thinness and funerals. But in the weeks that have followed, I feel the 'unwriterly' need to reject metaphors. To name things for what they are. Ducts and tumours and cells and lesions; facts, not fear. I am not 'fighting' cancer, because it is not a war. I am not 'surviving' it, at least no more than every human alive is 'surviving' life, the only certainty of which is death.

The edifice of modern medicine is pacifying. The hospital I go to is a private facility that specialises in cancer treatment. It reminds me somewhat of a small airport terminal. The registration front desk, down to the uniforms of the staff, is reminiscent of flight check-in. The nurses are like air hostesses, asking you to take a seat, and the doctors are like pilots telling you not to worry, it's just a bit of turbulence.

The place is always teeming. So many people with cancer: high society women and taciturn teenagers, the disoriented elderly and the tech bros who never seem to stop taking calls even as they are being wheeled away. Cancer patients are not a demographic, they are a microcosm of society.

These last few weeks, I've discovered just how cancerous the world is. Not a single person that I've shared my diagnosis with, has failed to tell me about an aunt, or mother, or best friend with the same disease. Others are 'survivors' themselves, although I hadn't known it.

But, lastly, the one question that has never occurred to me regarding the diagnosis, despite being a 46-year-old woman in reasonable health, is, 'Why me?' Because the real question is, 'Why not me?'

2

Living in the Present Moment

Yesterday is gone, tomorrow has not yet come. We have only today, let us begin.

—MOTHER TERESA

Living in the 'here and now' without being overwhelmed by the regrets of the past or the anxieties of the future has been prescribed as one of the best ways of coping with trauma.

This might appear impossible but it isn't really all that difficult. If we carefully look at a three-year-old child we can learn a lot about living in the moment. Whether the little one is drawing on a sheet of paper, or sailing a paper boat in a puddle or simply watching a bird in flight—she is giving her hundred percent to the present moment. She is not bothered about whether someone is watching her or laughing at her, she is not concerned about what she has done a few minutes earlier or what she is going to do a while later. We should all strive to adopt the natural, unselfconscious behaviour of the child and live life to the fullest.

In his book *Ichigo Ichie*, the bestselling author Hector Garcia writes, "In daily life, true meaning can be derived by living what a moment holds. When each moment is rich, life has no possibility of being any less than meaningful and satisfying. Just like the 16th Century Japanese tea ceremony where drinking tea was elevated to a slow ritual of wise consumption—*Ichigo Ichie* urges the reader to coax each moment of life to its inherent potential of fullness."

In her bestseller *The Human Side of Cancer*, Jimmie C. Holland MD emphasises that diagnosis of cancer brings with it both urgency as well as uncertainty. According to her the person who can say, "I'm just going to take one day at a time" is able to stay focussed on the tasks of the day. "I often remind people that you can't live yesterday or tomorrow, only today. Any big task seems overwhelming until you break it down into manageable parts. The Chinese say, 'You move a mountain by moving one stone at a time.' Hard as it is to keep thinking that way, coping with cancer is easier if you try not to focus on all the challenges that may lie ahead, but rather focus on today, during which you can accomplish something despite the problems caused by the treatment," she writes.

The following quote from Bhaddekaratta Sutta reflects this:

"Do not pursue the past.
Do not lose yourself in the future.
The past no longer is.
The future has not yet come.
Looking deeply at life as it is
in the very here and now,
the practitioner dwells
in stability and freedom."

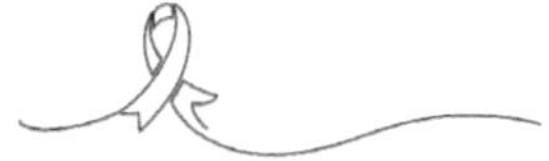

Case Study I: Surabhi Kakkar

Surabhi's husband Sunil was diagnosed with malignant tumour in his large intestine at a relatively young age of 41. Surabhi was shell shocked. But she soon realised she now had to look after her ailing husband, her six-year-old daughter and her elderly in-laws. She had to don the role of an anchor since her entire family now depended completely on her.

The period during which Sunil underwent treatment was the most harrowing one. But Surabhi did not give up. Throughout the entire ordeal she kept a smile on her face. Whenever negative thoughts intruded, she simply banished them and soldiered on.

Sharing her journey she writes, "Sunil's illness was a very traumatic time in our lives, but it really enforced our belief in the innate goodness of human nature. It bought to our focus the uncertainties of life. It made us sit up and rethink our goals. Our priorities changed and we also started appreciating and making the most of our time together, something we had started to take for granted earlier. I think the most important thing that I have learnt from the experience is that we cannot change the past, neither can we foresee the future, but today is a gift given to us to live fully, that is why it is called the present."

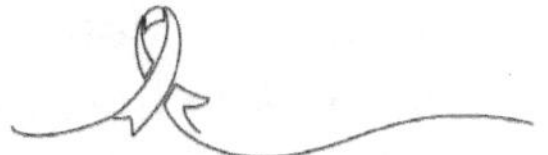

Case Study II: Vikram

Vikram, a cancer survivor, has been cancer free for some years now. However, the fear of recurrence continued to plague him.

He kept grappling with his fear for quite some time and then firmed up the following strategies to think of his past attainments, not worry about the future uncertainties and focus completely on the here and now:

> 'Separate the rational from the irrational:

  When I'm struggling with my emotional enemies, I try to remember how brave I have been and all the accomplishments I have had in my journey so far and I try to comfort myself through some positive affirmations.

> Fill your brain with positive thoughts:

  Focussing on the positives that I have witnessed in my healing journey also helps to filter the negative thoughts that continue popping up. I keep telling myself that life is what you make it.

> Allow the fear to move:

  When the emotion of fear is too strong, I don't let my mind carry me away with judgements and anxiety. I try to breathe-in and breathe-out and allow my mind to come back to the present moment. Sometimes this simple meditation makes my mind calm and I feel nourished.

> Use walking as a means to allay fear and anxiety:

  When I walk, my mind is fully in the walking body and each time I put my foot on the ground I am bringing my mind back to the present moment. This helps the tension to be released slowly. Being a little mindful can help us embrace our fears and strong emotions.'

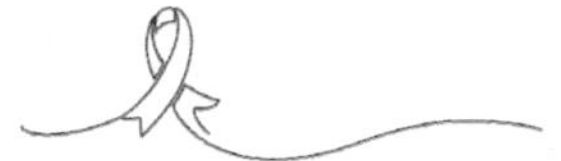

Case Study III: Jessica Reid Sliwerski

Jessica, the author of *Cancer Hates Kisses*, was diagnosed with breast cancer at a time in her life when she thought she could never be happier.

When she came to know about the disease she was completely devastated. She was continuously worried about the cancer spreading, about not making it during surgery, and about the disease recurring, even after doing everything she possibly could. She would fall asleep with fear clutching at her heart that she would not see her baby girl grow up.

Jessica goes on to describe how she came to appreciate the importance of each day and learnt to fight the terror of cancer—a journey which was tough, to say the least.

"One day during therapy, after unleashing a deluge of hypotheticals related to cancer, my therapist said in her soothing voice, 'All you can do is focus on today. Today the cancer is gone. Today you are doing chemo to kill everything else.'

Hearing this reminded me that as scary as cancer is, I am not powerless. Just as I had choices in my course of treatment, I have a choice now. I could continue to worry about all the things I cannot control and be depressed about the unfortunate fact that I had cancer, or I could choose to make each day a good day.... I could easily let the sadness of cancer cripple me, but instead I choose to rejoice in the gift of today.

Through these reframing exercises I have learned to suck every possible ounce of joy out of each day. As I told my therapist, 'I have accepted my cancer.' She corrected me, saying, 'No, you have embraced it'."

3

Normalising

I'm not bitter. Why should I be bitter? I'm thrilled to death with life.

—Johnny Cash, *American singer & song writer*

One of the common responses to the diagnosis of cancer is to treat it as the end of 'life as the person knew'. This is only partly true. As is seen from the many examples, there is life after cancer diagnosis and treatment, though it is a little different. An important aspect of coping is to bring 'normalcy' back to life, after the acute phase of treatment.

Normalising can be used as a coping strategy to make the illness part of one's daily life and not get overwhelmed by it. Here it will help to internalise the words of Robert Buckman, a cancer specialist, writer and TV personality: "Cancer is just a word, not a sentence."

In the following examples (adapted from *Existential Meaning-Making Coping in Iran*: A Qualitative Study among Patients with Cancer by F. Ahmadi *et al*), clear instances of this method can be seen:

In the first case, a 16-year-old young man, says: "I was very strong and I didn't let the disease overcome me. I believe that the fear of cancer is worse than cancer itself. Cancer was just a disease for me. I would continue my life. I played music. I watched movies. I didn't bother about the illness at all."

In the second case, a 75-year-old woman emphasised: "The disease is normal, if it's cured, great, if not, probably my life is finished, but I was not just sitting sadly and complaining that I'm dying. That is the worst thing one can do. If you give positive energy to yourself, you will receive the same, but if you feel defeated, you we will be defeated."

The third interviewee, a 28-year-old man, explained how he used normalising as a strategy: "Cancer or any other disease is a part of life, something that can happen and you shouldn't ask: 'Why should this happen to me?' In fact, getting cancer enriched my experiences. I would say this disease taught me to be more realistic."

Another case in point is the statement of a 35-year-old woman who said:

"After getting the diagnosis everything really became very beautiful for me…everything became enjoyable. With this new view, I began to live in a way so that if I die, I have no regrets and aspirations for me because I am full of pleasure and I have enjoyed everything around me."

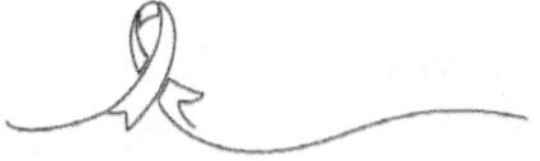

Case Study I: Sanjay Dutt

Bollywood superstar Sanjay Dutt was diagnosed with stage 4 lung cancer in August 2020 and was given only a 50 percent chance of survival.

The actor has a history of cancer in his family. He lost his mother Nargis Dutt and his wife Richa Sharma to cancer. He felt a sense of doom that he too wouldn't survive and his first reaction to the news was that he didn't want to go in for chemotherapy. If he was supposed to die, he would just die but wouldn't opt for any treatment.

However, he soon realised that his family was breaking down and he had to be strong for them. He decided to fight the illness and beat it.

According to his oncologist Dr. Sewanti Limaye, when Sanjay walked into her consultation room a week after the cancer diagnosis, he was calm and stoic.

"He had confronted his hour of reckoning and made a decision. He told me, 'I am going to go ahead as if I have never had cancer, just focus on getting my life back, breathe and follow whatever discipline is needed to do that.' Negativity was never an option for him. I would say he came with the most potent therapy there is: determination and willpower. And that's more than half the battle won."

Talking about the actor's journey, Dr. Limaye added, "His mental make-up was very strong, he never hid his illness and took the challenge head on from Day 1. He was open with his family and friends, wasn't scared to look weak in front of them, was honest with them and accepted their strength as and when required. That's the second most potent therapy there is, the support of family and friends, who can pull you out of troughs that any cancer therapy entails."

The star who epitomises guts and gumption in most of his movies exhibited the same courage during his cancer treatment. When the doctor warned him of losing hair and side effects like nausea, he said, *"Mereko kuch nahi hoga* (nothing will happen to me)." During chemotherapy when patients are usually crunched, he would spend two hours on the treadmill and even play badminton.

After being declared cancer free a few months after the diagnosis Sanjay Dutt said, "The last few weeks were very difficult for my family and me. But like they say, God gives the hardest battles to his strongest soldiers. And today, on the occasion of my kids' birthday, I am happy to come out victorious from this battle and be able to give them the best gift I can—the health and well-being of our family."

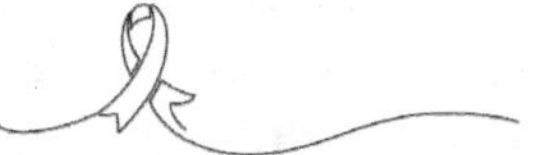

Case Study II: Neerja Chowdhury

Neerja Chowdhury, a brilliant journalist, was diagnosed with breast cancer in January 2002.

"Treat this as no more than a hiccup in the journey of life," a doctor friend advised her—a golden nugget which she internalised.

"Cancer is one of those words which arouse a sense of dread and virtually half kills a patient. I was fortunate in having a family who behaved normally. Otherwise, cancer can descend like a cloud over the family, affecting its spirit and functioning in myriad ways," she says.

The day Neerja got the report confirming the malignancy, she gritted her teeth and decided to keep the appointment with a politician. This she felt was her first step in treating the disease as little more than a blip. She decided early on that she wouldn't ask the question 'why me' to herself. Once she made the decision there was acceptance of the disease and within came a sense of peace.

"What also helped me cope was to go to work as usual, to write, to break stories as a journalist, to meet people, to push myself to keep a daily routine despite the listlessness which would often invade my body after the chemo injections. Sometimes, when I had a good story but was feeling tired and tempted to give up, in the office in the evening, my colleagues would say encouragingly, 'Just push it out somehow, and we will take care of cleaning up the copy'," she reminisces.

Neerja found that the surgery was not difficult and radiotherapy too was bearable. What made things a trifle easier was a simple advice (not by a doctor) that it would help to drink a whole bottle of water, even before she emerged out of the hospital, after a session of radiotherapy. The six cycles of chemotherapy, however, were a challenge. After the second injection, she came down with fever, cold, cough and bouts of vomiting. Whenever she would lie down, she would choke. As a result, she was terrified of lying down to sleep and would remain in the sitting position throughout the night. Her oncologist tweaked the quantum of medicine over the next four cycles so that her body could take it.

She had expected nausea to hit her the first day, but it did not. The effect of the first cycle lasted two days, and that of the last one, a whole week.

Neerja had been mentally ready for the loss of hair that would follow chemotherapy. But actually, when it started to happen, and shocks of hair started to come off, she was really not prepared for it.

"After my hair loss, a friend of mine based in London sent me a wig, which she got specially crafted for me (using my photograph), thinking it would help me look and feel 'normal'. But it was uncomfortable to wear in the hot weather and it was just not me. So, I took to wearing scarves on my head. But this meant a volley of questions, which I had to answer. Most people took it in a normal, natural way; only a few gave me the *bechari* look. Some journalist friends of mine naively thought I was trying to identify with Kashmiri women, when I went to Srinagar to write about the 2002 elections there!

Mercifully, when the hair grew back again after the treatment was over, it was a thicker growth, with a greater bounce. And I could opt for a new style!" she writes.

Through the difficult moments, Neerja kept reminding herself that the treatment and its after-effects would soon be behind her. At AIIMS, where she went for the first two rounds of chemotherapy, there was a poster hanging on the wall with the words, 'Do not forget, this too will pass'. It did.

She writes, "This may be a strange thing to say. In some ways, cancer came as a wake-up call for me, and gave me a new lease of life. Because cancer brings you so close to the possibility of death, you begin to sift the grain from the chaff, about what is important and what is not, with the realisation somewhere at the back of the mind that the clock might be ticking away. It was during one of those reflective moments one night that I decided that I must let go of the past burdens—the hurts and resentments—that had dogged my steps. It was almost like watching the baggage drift away.

My friends told me I began to look more alive. My colleagues told me that I was more prolific in the year of my treatment than in the previous years. It is wrong to say that cancer is a small happening. But it is easier to handle it, as I found, if you can accord it the import of 'only a hiccup in the journey of life'."

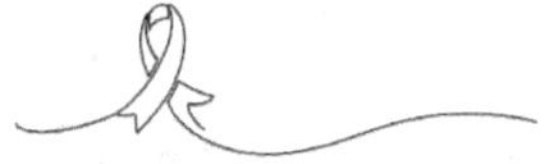

Case Study III: Ramen's experience

When my daughter Ankita was born, I made it clear to my wife Madhavi that I would not change her nappies (Ankita's nappies, fortunately Madhavi had far outgrown that stage!). I told my soul mate that I would, in every other way, care for our little bundle of joy. I would feed her, sing lullabies—though I admit, I am the second worst singer on Planet Earth (the worst, by far, being my father!)—I would give her a bath, tell her stories, dance to her gurgles... anything and everything except cleaning her poop. Crap completely grossed me out.

Who knew then that three decades later I would be wallowing in my own shit both figuratively and literally.

After my cancer diagnosis in November 2021, I underwent several cycles of radiation and chemotherapy. This was followed by the *daadi* of all surgeries (Colostomy) on 16th March 2022. I was decolonised—my colon (large intestine) was removed. The small intestine was brought out and a stoma bag was fitted to collect the faecal matter. Though the surgery took eight hours, there was no major issue and I was released from the hospital in three days. Since the doctors felt I had handled it like a champ they decided to go in for the Ileostomy closure on 6th April. This basically meant reconnecting the small intestine to the rectum and doing away with the stoma bag.

This was a much, much simpler operation but turned into a complete nightmare. Three septic shocks and two surgeries later I was back with the stoma bag. The 'crap collector' which I thought would be an itinerant visitor had returned like a prodigal—this time for keeps!

And, my unwanted guest was not a well-mannered boarder. It was a reckless profligate to say the least. The last two surgeries had resulted in a long and deep cut in the middle of my abdomen which took a long time to heal. As a result, the base plate of the stoma bag would get soggy due to the discharge from the adjacent surgery site and peel off and its 'precious' contents would spill all over.

Replacing the visitor with a new avatar, or to put it simply, changing the stoma bag needed professional expertise and we had to engage paramedical staff. Due to the traffic congestion and the distances in Bangalore, the nurse would take time to reach and I would be stuck with the muck.

The leakages continued randomly, and usually at the most inopportune moments. Even though I experimented with different types of em'body'ments, my body continued to 'settle' on my 'stool'. On some occasions the fault was the material (the quality of the bag), on others it was with the man (the nurse) but in the end, the trauma was all mine! I seemed to be drowning in my shit and 'owning' that of others.

In the initial stages even emptying the stoma bag was not easy. I was very weak and Madhavi had to help me out. After a while, I slowly learnt draining it on my own though I found the whole process disgusting. It was also mentally disturbing having the stoma bag always attached to me. It served, and still does, as a constant reminder of my, far from normal, condition.

I have been trying my best to get used to this new attachment, a tough task by any standards. I have to empty it around seven to eight times during the day and a couple of times at night. Since I am a very, very light sleeper I can sense when the bag is full and needs to be cleared. This, naturally, is a deterrent to proper sleep.

Necessity, it is said, is the mother of invention. I never found this cliché ring truer than when I started groping for solutions to managing my stoma bag.

I did a lot of research and zeroed in on an 'Ostomy Bath' apron. To my relief I found that the stoma bag fits quite snugly inside it. The apron is quite easy to wear and has enabled me to travel without the stress of the bag leaking. Of course, I did have to make a few adjustments of the sartorial kind. I can no longer tuck my shirt in. Either I wear it out or don a blazer, weather permitting of course. This is a small price to pay for the relief and the freedom. The 'Ostomy Bath' apron coupled with a tweaked wardrobe has helped me in keeping my trysts with storytelling and public speaking. I have even gone on stage and danced, and for a few evanescent moments, drained cancer out from my sensibilities just like I empty the stoma bag.

My son, Aniket, also indulged in some due diligence and bought me an Ostomy swimwear from Spain. I make sure my stoma bag fits cosily into it first, then wear my normal swimming costume over it. This way I have been able to swim, a passion which has provided emotional, mental and physical succour.

Another major breakthrough has happened, courtesy Madhavi. Over a period of time, she has learnt to replace the stoma bag. In fact, she does a far better job than the nurses. This has come as a huge relief. Now I no longer have to depend on an external agency and the vagaries of the weather and traffic snarls. Support is right beside me in the form of my 'love-in' partner!

So finally, after more than a year of 'sleeping with the enemy', I have succeeded in morphing the adversary into a Siamese twin who needs to be accepted and managed, not fought against or ignored.

4

Creating an Ecosystem of Positivity

Beautiful days do not come to you. You must walk towards them.

—Rumi

There is strong evidence for positivity decreasing distress and improving the illness outcome.

"Positivity can go a long way when you have been diagnosed with cancer, mine travelled so far, it had to get a visa!" quips Saranne Rothberg, who created 'The ComedyCures Foundation' from her chemo chair in 1999 and is still cancer-free.

Martin Seligman, a contemporary American psychologist, has done extensive work with positive psychology and what he calls as 'learned optimism' as a replacement to 'learned helplessness'.

"People start imagining the worst outcome which makes them fearful. Such a way of thinking is the hallmark of pessimism and can often lead to depression, compromise our immune system and have other adverse impacts on health. On the contrary, if someone looks at the possibility of occurrence of negative events in their least threatening fashion, as being temporary, as being conquerable, as challenges rather than threats then that disposition is called as optimistic style. The pessimists often attribute bad events as their own faults; believe that they are likely to happen; and that they have a permanency. While the optimists think that adverse happenings are confined only to a single case, that setback is not their fault and instead circumstances cause bad events to happen."

Seligman further says that optimism can be inculcated and learned just like any other skill. These skills help in shifting the paradigm from one of helplessness to one of greater personal control over fears. Helplessness is the 'giving up reaction' or the response to quit. While many things in life are beyond our control but many more are also within our control and our ability to fight fears is one such thing that is within our control. If we indulge in dwelling in our fears, we will find that they become self-fulfilling."

It is my personal belief that as effective as chemo, radiation and surgery—are our own willpower and resilience. Our most important goal should be to create an ecosystem of positivity.

Dr. Vijay Anand Reddy, Director of Apollo Cancer Institute, Hyderabad reiterates, "The importance of staying positive from day one of your diagnosis cannot be over-emphasised. It has been scientifically proven that a patient with a positive attitude is more likely to survive. He or she will experience fewer side effects and recover faster. By all means expect the worst and be prepared to face it, but do not lose your optimism."

As Karen Salmansohn, the well-known self-help book author and designer says, "You gotta look for the good in the bad, the happy in your sad, the gain in your pain, and what makes you grateful not painful."

Being positive will not make your life longer but it will make each moment you live more enriching and fulfilling.

Don't wait for the light at the end of the tunnel to reach you. Rush ahead, grab it, pull it forward till it becomes one with you. Remember once you start creating an ecosystem of positivity the entire universe will come together to offer you succour, solace and strength.

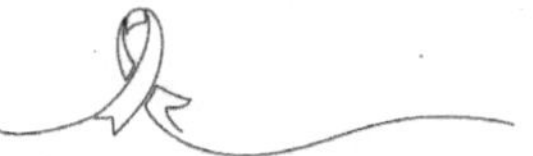

Case Study I: Manisha Koirala

Manisha Koirala has played diverse roles in Indian films winning both popular and critical acclaim.

She was diagnosed with stage 4 ovarian cancer in November 2012 and was declared cancer free after a tough fight in April 2013. The most critical part of the treatment was her surgery at Sloan-Kettering Hospital in New York.

Manisha reminisces about the time she spent in the Big Apple. "I chose to be with and listen to only positive people. My friend Zakia told me how her sister coped with it. She said, 'Don't call it chemo but a vitamin shot.' On Lisa Ray's blog, I read that she had a chemo cut which was a bald look. I felt it was a great attitude to have. Everybody had a mechanism to deal with it. They had a certain twang or twist which made it sound fun or spunky. There were also people who psych you out by saying 'Chemo is poison and it's going to go in your bloodstream and you are going to die'. They scare you even more. I chose to be away from them."

What were the life lessons cancer taught her? "Through this ordeal I know how uncertain life is now. For all these years I thought I could live longer until cancer hit me. After it, I realise how fragile it is. But my life doesn't end with the cancer story. It happened, I dealt with it, if it happens again, I will deal with it again and move on.

The fear exists. But I don't get victimised by it. I have no other choice but to live with it. The maximum fear is that I'm going to die or have a painful death. I don't panic about it anymore. There is no bitterness about the experience. I am happier and content."

According to the actress, cancer had a huge impact on her perspective towards life. It made her kinder, gentler and taught her that 'we are all interconnected and intertwined'.

"I literally started seeing joy in small things like walking on the grass, the breeze on my face, looking out of my bed at the sky and clouds, sunsets and sunrises—I started noticing small things, because tomorrow I didn't know whether I would be alive to see it. Everything is new to me. I value everything more including human beings. I feel like giving hugs to people *chalte chalte*."

Manisha's advice to cancer patients is clear and concise.

"When I was diagnosed with cancer, I was shattered and devastated. But I was quick to understand that this was like any other disease, and I had to fight it out. Besides family support, which is very important, I feel that patients should understand the responsibility of handling it by themselves! They should follow the doctor's advice diligently, take care of their nutrition, maintain good hygiene and fight with a positive attitude." *Touché*!

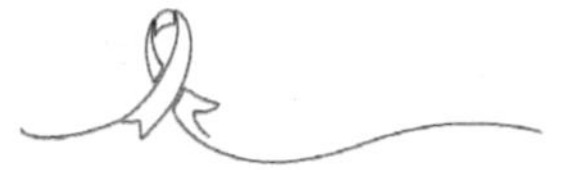

Case Study II: Tanisa Dhingra

On 8th March 2016, Tanisa was diagnosed with stage 3 metastatic ovarian cancer, only a few months short of her 23rd birthday. After battling with rare courage and positivity, for more than five years, she succumbed to the disease.

Even as Tanisa was fighting the dreaded disease she wrote, "Cancer stormed into my life back in 2016 and took me by storm. But as they say 'Nothing can hurt you without your permission' so I didn't let it break me. As part of my recovery, I had to move to USA during this phase and I made so many memories out of the most challenging time, by making friends at the most uncommon places and travelling my heart out. It made me a new person. I wanted to make a significant difference to society and bring awareness that life is beyond my disease, it is in moments you miss out on living.

I want people to detoxify from the word 'Cancer' and look at it from a new perspective. It's a difficult journey, but it should not pull you down.

I say—keep it real! Keep it moving! If you are someone who knows how to flaunt your 'real' in the toughest of times, you are doing justice to your story."

Tanisa was advised several sessions of chemotherapy followed by a surgery to remove the orange-sized tumour. She then underwent some more sessions of chemo.

"Having no prior exposure to or knowledge about something so far-reaching made me fear the big 'C' even more. Before I could even comprehend the gravity of the situation, the therapy began."

Tanisa decided to take the road less travelled because that was her only option. It made her a strong-willed person, taught her gratitude, grit and the essence and importance of life. Tanisa wanted to make it easier for her parents to deal with the news by being their source of strength even when she herself was at the weakest.

"I'm an inherently happy person, you see. The kind of person who smiles across to you from afar, a genuine smile. I wanted to preserve that. I would be lying if I said there were no bad days, there were plenty. But I'd cry it out, take my painkillers, ride my Scooty, binge on amazing American cuisine and tour across the USA.

My journey continues to teach me something daily through small incidents and that is what I wish to write about and share with the world. I encountered the nicest people and this is my way of trying to acknowledge and reinforce people's faith in humanity."

In the five years after being diagnosed with ovarian cancer, Tanisa managed to spread not just immense joy but also helped thousands of others break free of the stigma that cancer carries. She provided financial aid wherever needed and helped patients rediscover life post-cancer.

The first reaction of Tanisa's mother Meenakshi Dhingra to the catastrophic news was of complete disbelief—she went into a denial mode.

"When I came to know about my daughter's diagnosis, I was shell shocked. The doctor was saying something but I couldn't hear properly. I thought the hospital has committed a blunder. This cannot be true. How can someone so young and healthy have this disease? A person who takes utmost care of her diet, has a near perfect lifestyle and exercises regularly...how can she fall prey to cancer? I went back to the Radiologist and asked if there had been a mistake—had Tanisa's report been exchanged with someone else's?"

However, when the horrific news was confirmed Meenakshi and her husband Neeraj took Tanisa to USA for treatment, which lasted for a year. The responsibility of handling their flourishing export business was given to their office staff. Their younger son who had just commenced his class XII board exams was left in the care of Meenakshi's mother who herself was unwell.

Meenakshi and Neeraj had to face huge challenges. They were in a completely new space where everything including the healthcare system was alien. They had neither financial nor emotional support and had to figure out everything on their own. The biggest trauma was watching their young and vibrant daughter caught in the throes of a dreaded disease.

Tanisa and her family fought strongly and she was into remission the same year. She however had a relapse in 2020, and after a long and hard battle, she passed away on 30th December 2021.

When asked about her advice to caregivers Meenakshi says, "Frankly speaking, there cannot be any advice since each caregiver will have his/her our own coping mechanisms. No matter how strong you feel, you will have different emotions at different moments. There will be times when things become unbearable but as a caregiver you have to be strong for your loved ones."

However, she has a few generic tips for those who are around the patients in their most challenging times:

➢ Remain positive when you are with the patient no matter what the doctors say.

➢ Giving up is not an option.

- ➤ Read/watch inspirational stories.
- ➤ Have faith in your faith.
- ➤ Take some time out for yourself every day. Spend that time praying, meditating or pursuing a hobby.
- ➤ Take turns with your family members. Everyone doesn't have to be around always.
- ➤ Be with people who are positive. Cut yourself off from the Cassandras.
- ➤ Look after yourself. Only if you are fit will you be able to take care of your loved ones.

After losing Tanisa, Meenakshi Dhingra set up a Foundation to help improve cancer care in India—something her daughter always wanted to do. The foundation has benefited over 2,500 cancer survivors so far.

5

Connecting with the Self

You cannot teach a man anything; you can only help him find it within himself.

—Galileo Galilei

All illnesses bring back the attention to the self, as everything has to be experienced by the individual.

In the paper 'Existential Meaning-Making Coping in Iran: A Qualitative Study among Patients with Cancer', the researchers emphasise that connecting with the self is a defence mechanism and is essentially about how an individual sees himself and his personal and social roles.

To explain this mechanism, they quote a 22-year-old man: "I say that I rely on myself and myself alone in this world and do not depend on anything or anybody. I know that if I want and try, I will win and get what I want. I know that whatever would happen in my life, it could not be as difficult as this disease, and it was this disease that made me believe that I could overcome the other difficulties in the future… This disease taught me how to deal with the problems of life. And in the meantime, my inner power made me believe that I would recover, and I believed these conditions were not lasting, and that everything would not end here and life would continue."

In this case the young man connects with his inner self and copes with the disease through his strong will to live.

The research quotes another individual, a 35-year-old woman, who faces the malady by controlling everything in her life, "I have controlled my entire life so far and I have almost done everything I wanted and I do not need anyone… I hate my life as a routine. I enjoyed my period of illness because I was in a position where I could prove to myself and others that they are thinking in the wrong way about many things. I want to find a world that's worth keeping anyway."

These two individuals exemplify how by connecting with the self and drawing strength from what is within even the toughest of situations can be faced.

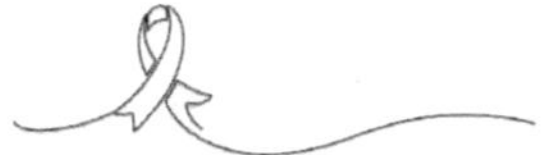

Case Study I: Irrfan Khan

Irrfan Khan was one of Bollywood's most acclaimed stars who achieved considerable success in British and American cinema as well.

He was diagnosed with Neuroendocrine cancer and spoke about his mindset in an interview to *The Times of India* on 18th June 2018.

"It's been quite some time now since I have been diagnosed with a high-grade neuroendocrine cancer. This new name in my vocabulary, I got to know, was rare, and due to fewer study cases, and less information comparatively, the unpredictability of the treatment was more. I was part of a trial-and-error game.

I had been in a different game, I was travelling on a speedy train ride, had dreams, plans, aspirations, goals, was fully engaged in them. And suddenly someone taps on my shoulder and I turn to see. It's the TC: 'Your destination is about to come. Please get down.'

I am confused: 'No, no. My destination hasn't come.'

'No, this is it. This is how it is sometimes.'

The suddenness made me realise how you are just a cork floating in the ocean with UNPREDICTABLE currents! And you are desperately trying to control it.

In this chaos, shocked, afraid and in panic, while on one of the terrifying hospital visits, I blabber to my son, 'The only thing I expect from ME is not to face this crisis in this present state. I desperately need my feet. Fear and panic should not overrule me and make me miserable.'

That was my INTENTION. AND THEN THE PAIN HIT. As if all this while, you were just getting to know pain, and now you know its nature and its intensity. Nothing was working; NO consolation, no motivation. The entire cosmos becomes one at that moment—just PAIN, and pain felt more enormous than GOD."

As he was entering the hospital, drained, exhausted, listless, Irrfan hardly noticed that his hospital was on the opposite side of Lord's, the stadium. The Mecca of his childhood dream. Amidst the pain, he saw a poster of a smiling Vivian Richards. Nothing happened, as if that world didn't ever belong to him.

This hospital also had a coma ward right above Irrfan's room. One day while he was standing on the balcony, the peculiarity jolted him. He realised that between the game of life and the game of death, there was just a road. On one side was the hospital, on the other, a stadium. He realised that he wasn't part of anything which might claim certainty—neither the hospital, nor the stadium.

He was left with the immense effect of the enormous power and intelligence of the cosmos. The uniqueness of his hospital's location slammed into Irrfan. He comprehended that the only thing certain was the uncertainty. All he could do was to actualise his strength and play his game better.

As he said, "This realisation made me submit, surrender and trust, irrespective of the outcome, irrespective of where this takes me, eight months from now, or four months from now, or two years. The concerns took a backseat and started to fade and kind of went out of my mind space.

For the first time, I felt what 'freedom' truly means. It felt like an accomplishment. As if I was tasting life for the first time, the magical side of it. My confidence in the intelligence of the cosmos became absolute. I feel as if it has entered every cell of mine.

Time will tell if it stays, but that is how I feel as of now.

Throughout my journey, people have been wishing me well, praying for me, from all over the world. People I know, people I don't even know. They were praying from different places, different time zones, and I feel all their prayers become ONE. One big force, like a force of current, which got inside me through the end of my spine and has germinated through the crown of my head.

It's germinating—sometimes a bud, a leaf, a twig, a shoot. I keep relishing and looking at it. Each flower, each twig, each leaf which has come from the cumulative prayers, each fills me with wonder, happiness and curiosity.

A realisation that the cork doesn't need to control the current. That you are being gently rocked in the cradle of nature."

Irrfan Khan passed away on 29th April 2020 from a colon infection caused by the disease.

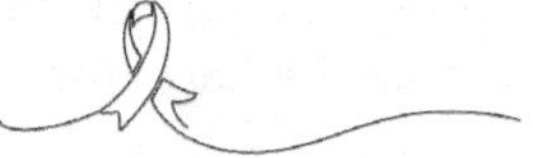

Case Study II: Neena Singh

Neena Singh is a breast cancer survivor of more than two decades.

"The journey from 'I have breast cancer' to 'I am leading a normal life' has undoubtedly been very long and arduous. Every morning when I stuffed cotton in my bra to get dressed my eyes would fill up with tears. Why this had to happen to me? Yes, there have been worries and low self-esteem and tears too… Slowly, I discovered that it was not the physical but emotional wounds that proved more difficult to heal. But one gets through life step by step, one day at a time. I wake up every morning and thank God that I am alive. I am still there for my daughters, husband and, of course, me."

Neena always goes back to what her oncologist told her, "You can wake up each morning and worry about dying, or you can wake up each morning and celebrate living."

She has realised that there is life after cancer and has worked towards making it a good life. She is not defined by the disease. She lives one day at a time and values each and every day.

"Cancer has changed my life for the better. We are a much closer family now than we were before. I don't worry about details which are not important."

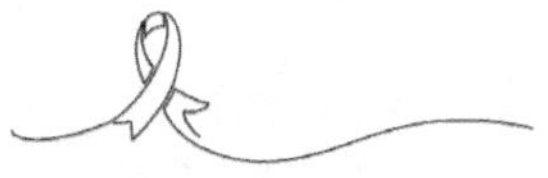

Case study III: Marilyn French

Marilyn French is an American radical feminist author who was diagnosed with oesophageal cancer. Her experience as a cancer survivor was the basis for her book *A Season in Hell: A Memoir*.

French talks about how after the verdict of cancer she connected with herself and redefined and redesigned her life.

"I no longer have large scale desires. I no longer wish for or expect undying love, perfect harmony within my family, a life in which everything is right (which, however absurd it may be, I did desire and kept anticipating before). I have only small desires—for a glass of cold orange juice, a good book, a visit with someone I love. Not only do I have no large desires for myself; I no longer have them for the world. . . It destroyed my absurd and unconscious belief that because I could see the ideal, I had the responsibility to help others see it, to create it. The weight of this responsibility was heavy, and carrying it made me angry. . . .

Coming close to death as I did engraved on my consciousness the understanding that the ideal is not going to happen, that it was always a delusion, the daydream of a wilful child. . . I am no longer driven. . . I am free. I am permitted to enjoy myself. I have noticed that my laugh has changed, is more spontaneous, deeper. I am almost serene. I cannot say that I am happy that I was sick, but that I am happy that sickness, if it had to happen, brought me to where I am now. It is a better place than I have been before. I am grateful to have been allowed to live long enough to experience it."

6

Investing in Relationships

Connecting with those you know love, like and appreciate you restores the spirit and gives you energy to keep moving forward in this life.

—Deborah Day, *Author of Be Happy Now*

In the rodent race called life we often forget to forge relationships.

Dr. Rashmi H.R. in her book *Holistic Happy You* stresses on the importance of building strong bonds. "We are made to interact and connect with others. Without meaningful relationships, we are lonely and isolated. We're happier when we pursue happiness with others. Find the right people to be associated with. Hang out with happy people as moods are contagious and feelings can be transferred from one to another."

Many of us are so busy getting stuff for our loved ones by investing money that we forget to give something which is free but invaluable—the gift of a memory. We should realise that memories do not get obsolete; they last a lifetime, like diamonds they are forever.

"When news of her cancer first broke, I had neither the wisdom nor the perspective, but I saw it clearly now. God did have a purpose in all of this. My time with *Amma*, these six weeks, felt like a special gift, delivered straight from heaven. Watching the same soap operas, I had earlier yawned through, movies and music shows I had not cared for, *Amma* and I were filling a fresh bank of precious memories," says Padma (name changed), a caregiver to her mother.

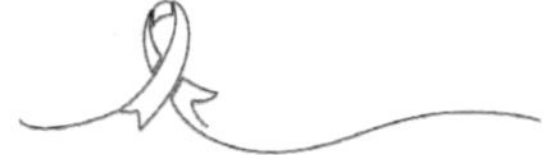

Case Study I: Ramen's experience

We have all heard of an ATM card or Automatic Teller Machine card. I would like to share the concept of a new ATM card—the Any Time Memory Card. How is this currency created? By investing in two four letter words—Love and Time. What makes this card so special? It cannot be lost, stolen, damaged or hacked. It is not plastic; it is for real. It has no value, simply because it is priceless. And above all it has no expiry date.

As my children Ankita and Aniket were growing up, I made conscious, deliberate efforts at creating memories—to leave behind a legacy of endearing moments for them. Every year during the first burst of rain which usually happens in the month of May, we used to go out on the lawn in front of our house. There in broad daylight, clad in our shorts, we got totally drenched. As we waded through the slush and mud, singing and dancing to glory, the moments were captured on camera. This unselfconscious, uninhibited and unadulterated madness went on for years.

When the kids were still quite young, together we also evolved the concept of 'Papa's Day Out'.

My wife Madhavi would be packed off to office for the day. After attaining 'freedom', the three of us would go berserk. The entire agenda would be set by the kids.

We would dress up in wacky clothes, go to the local zoo, gobble up street food and watch nutty movies. In fact, we would end up doing anything and everything which was loony.

When the Corona Virus was in full rampage, our family of five (including our lab, Aryan) was closeted together for three months. All four humans were working from home. This was the first time we were together in 12 years and that too confined within four walls—with nowhere to go. I was thinking, two overgrown teens in their twenties and two immature adults in their fifties—how would we manage without tearing each other apart!

But we did and how! What we indulged in was a simple trick—encashing our respective ATM cards. And once we did that, out came a virtual avalanche of memories—each more delectable than the other.

We would bring out the photo albums and laugh and drool at every picture and the delightful reminiscence behind it. The magic carpet of memories took us not to unknown lands but to very familiar, very comfortable cocoons which we had not revisited for years!

Everyone was fighting Covid by maintaining social distancing, wearing masks and washing hands. Our family was battling Covid by bridging emotional distances, wearing smiles and tugging at memories.

During the terrible cancer ordeal too our ATM cards came to our rescue. The indelible connect we shared, glued together by our endearing and enduring memories, helped us navigate through the worst turbulence of our lives.

Here I would like to share my tribute to Madhavi who played Savitri to my Satyavan at every step of my fight with the deadly malady. Our relationship defined by trust, mutual respect and unconditional commitment was the elixir that saved me.

MY 'ROCK'ING ANGEL

As I lay, down and almost out
In the isolation ICU,
My senses totally smothered
And my entire body almost blue.

The doctors had given up
Having tried their best,
But to you I was life itself
Not an itinerant guest.

Before we had lived our dreams
How could you let me go?
I was your forever bestie
In every high and low.

You gave me your strength
You virtually took on death,
With the weapon of your faith
You battled for my every breath.

You fought many a battle
Won for me many a war,
Nursing my every wound
And healing my every scar.

Now as I march steadfast
On the path of recovery
With you, my 'Rock'ing angel
The epitome of bravery.

I thank the Lord above
For making you mine
And giving you the courage
That is truly sublime.

When I look around and see
Lives which are in a tangle,
I know my Life is safe
With you my 'Rock'ing Angel.

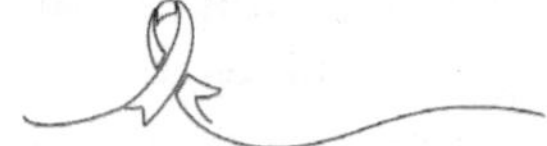

Case Study II: Pallavi Aiyar

Pallavi is an award-winning journalist and author. She was diagnosed with cancer in August 2022 and lost her mother Gitanjali Aiyar, well known Doordarshan anchor of yesteryears, in June 2023.

Pallavi believes that her cancer diagnosis hit her mother harder than it hit her. Gitanjali spent one month with Pallavi's family which was staying in Spain.

During that period, Gitanjali was reading a book on the technical/practical aspects of breast cancer. In the book she found a section on tips to get through the early days of a diagnosis that included a suggestion to start a 'jar of joy'.

The idea was for the cancer patient to write notes to herself every time she experienced a micro-joy (birds singing or a particularly tight hug from a child) and to put these in a jar. These could then be returned when the patient felt low. According to Pallavi this little advice was guaranteed to put a smile on even the most chemo-fatigued face.

During her sojourn in Spain, Pallavi's younger son, 11-year-old Nico and Gitanjali started writing and collecting notes in his school notebook. They called it the 'Book of Memories'.

Back home after her mom's death, Pallavi went back to reading and re-reading the book as a part of her healing journey and saw it with a completely fresh perspective. "What she had written for me to cope with a mastectomy and lymphadenectomy, I now saw in a new light—as her goodbye messages, leaving behind something I will cherish forever. Each message still gives me goosebumps. I am not a spiritual person but this felt cosmic. Mumma and I shared an unusually close relationship; however, being close also means that we tend to take the person for granted. It's funny how we reserve our best behaviour for others, while our close ones get to see the unfiltered side of ours. My mother however was very patient with me, always loving and she would never hold it against me—instead, she would just absorb it all. I want to be that with my kids. The book of memories has reminded me that there are several small and important joys that we must cherish, every single day."

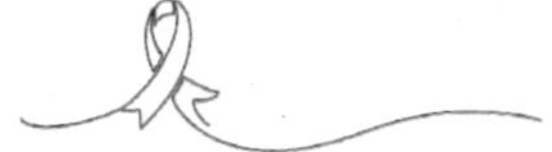

Case Study III: Sunaina

Sunaina passed away just 10 days before her 58th birthday. She suffered from gastrointestinal stromal tumour (GIST) cancer for close to three years. It is one of the most debilitating and painful diseases, aggressively attacking the entire body and the mind too. She was never admitted to any hospital, was at home throughout except for regular check-ups. Hence care was arranged at home. Towards the last few months, she rapidly lost weight, her appetite was impacted and she had to be goaded to eat like a child. Her bones began to protrude but fortunately her mind was alert even up to the last 3–4 days.

Sunaina decided not to return to the US, where she used to reside, shifting to Chandigarh to stay with her mother who was in her seventies. This meant adjustments, both on her part as well as her son's who had to shift too. Her sister Sujata who was living in another city took leave frequently from her office to spend time with Sunaina. Other members of the family and friends chipped in as well.

Spending time, socialising, going out, talking, laughing and being normal helped. The family organised get-togethers, parties, went walking in the beautiful parks of Chandigarh. Sunaina even came for a family wedding to Delhi despite being in poor health. She was excited like a child throughout—meeting everyone and participating in all the functions. She arranged a surprise party on Sujata's birthday even though she was bed ridden.

Sujata writes, "Please understand that a person who is sick has emotional upheavals. Do not take things personally. Very often they become more blunt, aggressive, short-tempered. It's important to express your love to them and forget the differences, if any. Also mend broken bridges to the extent possible."

7

Finding a Sense of Purpose

Twenty years from now you will be more disappointed by the things that you didn't do than by the ones you did do. So, throw off the bowlines. Sail away from the safe harbour. Catch the trade winds in your sails. Explore. Dream. Discover.

—MARK TWAIN

The diagnosis of cancer, for many patients, brings with it a whole range of emotions—from helplessness to hopelessness, anger, agony, angst and grief. They are suddenly faced with humongous challenges related to the physical condition, work, family, finances, stigma and above all the trauma of tomorrow. Even if many of these issues are taken care of by family and friends, life to many becomes meaningless. They feel they are a burden to the family and society. Their existence becomes hollow. In this situation finding a sense of purpose becomes critical.

A mission or a vision which gives them a sense of worth, which helps them actualise their feelings becomes the lodestar that can guide them forward.

"Self-absorption in all its forms kills empathy, let alone compassion. When we focus on ourselves, our world contracts as our problems and preoccupations loom large. But when we focus on others, our world expands. Our own problems drift to the periphery of the mind and so seem smaller, and we increase our capacity for connection—or compassionate action," says Daniel Goleman, the author of the seminal *Emotional Intelligence*.

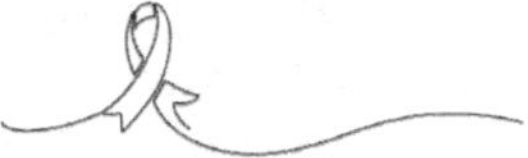

Case Study I: Brigadier SC Sharma

Brigadier SC Sharma was diagnosed with cancer of the food pipe on 20th October 1994. He underwent a major surgery followed by chemotherapy which led to a heart attack. He then had to undergo radiotherapy and the prognosis was that he wouldn't survive more than three months. After a hiatus he had to undergo another surgery to remove an obstruction in the intestine. By then he was aware that there was 80 percent chance of the recurrence of cancer within the first five years. He retired from service in 1996 and devoted his life to helping people battling with cancer.

Thus, the Brigadier found his sense of purpose in altruism.

"It is my firm belief that true happiness lies in giving. Giving can take many forms; it can be a smile, a handshake, or offering a caring word or sympathetic listening. The famous American TV host Oprah Winfrey once remarked, 'Giving is not about being able to write a cheque, but being able to touch someone's life'. It goes without saying that altruism and social involvement infuse a warmth and glow that relieve stress and promote longevity," the Brigadier says.

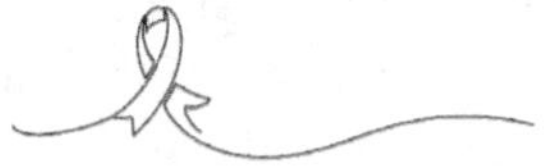

Case study II: Asha Choudhry

Asha Choudhry was detected with breast cancer in February 1996. Six months later she had to undergo mastectomy. Six cycles of chemotherapy and 25 rounds of radiation followed. Due to the aggressive treatment regimen of three months, medicines and injections, she lost all her hair, her skin turned black and looked charred. She was physically and emotionally drained and lost the will to live.

After her treatment she joined a cancer support group and soon there was a paradigm shift in her outlook. "My depression slowly took a backseat and I felt inspired to do something to alleviate the suffering and trauma of cancer patients. I realised the need to rise above my personal grief and devote my time and energy in providing emotional support to other cancer-afflicted patients.

Many years down the line, I look back and feel satisfied that I have brought some cheer in the lives of some people and given them the courage to fight. I see myself as a missionary with a mission to spread the light of hope to dispel the darkness generated by the diagnosis of cancer. My work has given me a new purpose and meaning to my life. I shall continue my work till the last breath," says Asha.

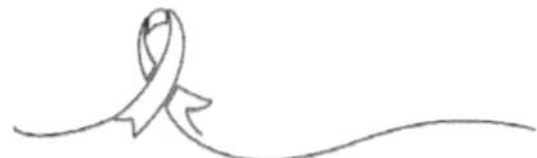

Case Study III: Prerna

Prerna's mother Arti (name changed) was diagnosed with breast cancer on 8th June 2014 at the age of 64. Till then she had enjoyed good health and a fulfilling life. She received the diagnosis with great poise and gave the family the courage to go ahead with her treatment.

Her mastectomy was done within two weeks of her diagnosis. The surgery was followed by six courses of chemotherapy. Each of these courses was 21 days apart. After chemo she had to undergo three weeks of radiation therapy.

Arti took the initial treatment in her stride. However, as it progressed, she began getting depressed. The family did its best to make her comfortable and let her rest. This turned out to be a blunder. She had always been the pivot around which the family had revolved. Caring and cooking were her main roles which she was now being deprived of. She began to feel that she was useless and would not be loved anymore.

Prerna realised the grave mistake the family had committed by doing 'everything' for her mother. She understood that most of the individuals value themselves on the basis of their 'usefulness' to others.

Prerna started making all out efforts to involve her mother in the activities she had loved doing before her illness—cooking, cleaning and caring.

Soon she found Arti taking over all the household responsibilities and becoming lively and cheerful once again.

"I strongly believe that the restoration of her sense of purpose did aid her speedy recovery. The purpose of life of individuals depends on their values and life experiences. My mother's purpose in life was to be the ultimate caregiver. She hated finding herself at the receiving end. It is very important for us caregivers to understand that our loved ones do not need our sympathy what they want is our empathy," Prerna reiterates.

8

Building Resilience

A scar does not form on the dying. A scar means I survived.
—Chris Cleave, *British writer & Journalist*

In the research article 'Wellbeing: Through the Lens of Indian Traditional Conceptualisations' Venkat R. Pulla and K.K.K. Salagame write that according to Indian tradition, resilience or 'Abhyâsa' is a spiritual practice that is defined by people's capacity to cope with loss, grief and insurmountable odds.

"When people enhance their strengths and resources and work towards overcoming obstacles, they become resilient. This resilience in turn generates optimism and hope. Hope for many may be an impossible dream, but for those who are resilient, it is the only possible step to take to continue a purposeful life," they reiterate.

In the paper 'Existential Meaning-Making Coping in Iran: A Qualitative Study among Patients with Cancer' the researchers have mentioned studies which have revealed that the painful journey cancer patients undergo can bring about 'A turning point'—a new positive attitude towards life. They have quoted a 22-year-old man: "I learned to deal with hardship and used its positive aspects to continue my life, because I believe that when it comes to one's life, experiences can be beneficial. It's not important how difficult the situations are, the personality growth caused by these harsh situations is important and valuable. If anyone understands this, (s)he can rebuild a new life on this basis."

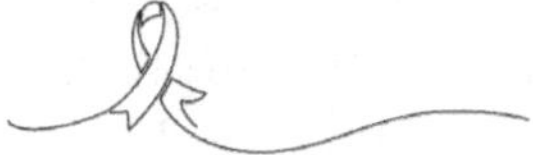

Case study I: Yuvraj Singh

Yuvraj Singh is an international cricketing legend who played a pivotal role in India's victories in the 2007 ICC World Twenty20 and the 2011 Cricket World Cup.

In November 2011, it was reported that Yuvraj was suffering from a tumour in his lung. Three months later, it was confirmed it was malignant and that he had mediastinal seminoma—a rare type of lung cancer.

It is hard to believe that Yuvraj had been suffering right through the World Cup. In fact, the ordeal had begun even before the ICC event. He was vomiting blood during India's tour of South Africa in January 2011. The agony and fatigue got worse by the time the World Cup started.

"At first I was in denial about it—playing for India was more important than my health and for a few months I chose to ignore the blood I spat out or my decline in stamina," says the cricketing icon.

The fact that he put up such a stellar show leading India to an incredible victory and winning the player of the tournament award, even while fighting the demon of cancer, speaks volumes for his incredible willpower.

Shabnam Singh, Yuvraj's mother recalls that she went completely numb the moment she came to know about her son's cancer. It gradually sunk in but it took her a long time to come to terms with the fact.

Yuvraj had to undergo three intensive chemotherapy sessions in the US.

Regarding the challenging time she and Yuvraj went through, Shabnam says, "The doctor told us that the treatment was going to be very difficult but that Yuvraj would be cured and that he would be able to start playing again after six weeks of therapy. It was wonderful to hear the doctor say that and I clung onto that piece of news. We had also read Lance Armstrong's book where he had mentioned that the treatment was very harsh, it would make you miserable and you would start crying for no reason. So, when I saw Yuvraj crying, I would only think that the medicine was working rather than thinking why my son was crying."

Yuvraj has huge admiration for his mother's grit and resilience—qualities he believes are epitomised by all caregivers.

"Whenever my pain became unbearable during the treatment, my mother was there as a pillar of strength. Not for a moment did she give up hope for my complete recovery and that gave me the willpower to fight cancer. So, I strongly believe that caregivers are a strong source of support during the treatment process. I salute them for their unbelievable courage and perseverance during their loved one's long and tedious journey towards recovery."

Shabnam echoes the very same sentiment, "If the caregiver gets emotional and starts crying in front of the patient, then the patient also gets weak. I would panic sometimes, especially once when he fainted in my arms, but I never cried in front of Yuvraj. In fact, whenever he cried, I just held him and said you are going to be fine. If I had also gone weak, how could I have given the strength to my son to fight the disease? To give strength to the cancer patient and to motivate him or her is the role of the caregiver. Halfway through his treatment, Yuvraj knew that he could either cry about it or be strong about it. He decided to be strong and that's how he came out of it."

When Yuvraj heard the word cancer for the first time, he got terribly scared. Cancer was like a death sentence. He became really unsure where life would take him. It was only when he accepted cancer that he could beat it. He kept himself motivated throughout his tough journey.

As he says, "When life knocks you down you have a choice—to get up. No matter how difficult it gets, don't give up."

It is noteworthy that after his recovery Yuvraj returned to cricket in 2012 and continued playing at the highest level before retiring in 2017.

So, how has his fight with cancer changed Yuvraj? "Once you have a close encounter with death, you realise the real value of life. Simple things like breathing, enjoying food, the small pleasures of life that we take for granted, become precious. The bodily suffering, when I was choking while trying to breathe, when I couldn't digest anything each time I had chemo, when I would be a mental and physical wreck, made me realise that living a normal life is a blessing and should not be frittered away by fretting over things which are beyond your control."

After winning their personal battle against cancer, Yuvraj and his mother founded the YouWeCan Foundation in 2012 as a non-profit organisation. Its objective is to eradicate the stigma around cancer, create awareness about the need for early detection as well as support underprivileged cancer patients during and after their treatment.

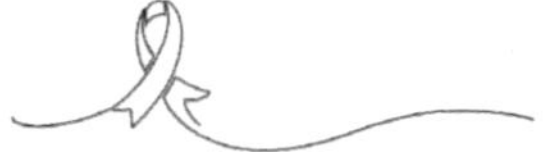

Case Study II: Dr. Sudesh Mukhopadyaya

Dr. Sudesh Mukhopadyaya was diagnosed during routine medical check-up with Breast Cancer in early August, 2016 with tumour at Grade III and cancer at stage II A. Within a week all tests indicated the urgency for surgery.

Mastectomy was performed and she braved the surgery and the loss of a breast with her innate will power.

She had to undergo 16 rounds of chemo with the first two posing daunting challenges. She lost her hair and the doctors advised her to get a wig. However, she decided to see how Nature would redesign her.

She also lost weight, suffered continuous fever and had to undergo several rounds of hospitalisation and blood transfusion. But by the third chemo onwards, thanks to her intrinsic resilience and the humongous support of her family and friends, she healed quickly.

She is now back to living life with a new hairstyle, a clear skin and above all a glowing enthusiasm to do her best till her last breath.

"I have learnt that Life is never a straight line; it has all its curves and plateaus. It is for us to traverse these paths and accept life as it evolves and live it to the fullest," Dr. Sudesh says.

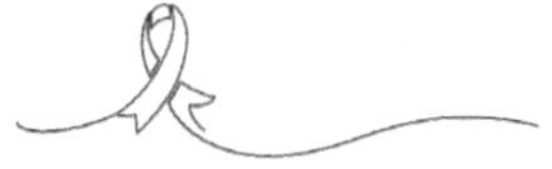

Case Study III: Manish Mittal

Manish Mittal's daughter Mansi was diagnosed with blood cancer when she was at the tender age of 20 months. Manish and his wife, who was pregnant at that time, were completely shattered by the horrifying news.

When the chemotherapy treatment started Manish found it unbearable to watch Mansi undergo the torture. "Watching your toddler go through chemotherapy is one of the most painful things a parent can endure. You know that the chemo is important for your child to recover, but seeing her suffer from the side-effects is most painful. Each time I watched the neon red liquid enter her veins, I sat there next to her on the hospital bed, wondering if I could have prevented her suffering in any way. I keep wondering whether there could have been some neglect on my part that caused my child to develop leukaemia. The doctors have explained to me many times that it is not because of anything we did, that cancer can affect anyone. The reasons for this are not fully known to us yet. But still, as a parent, I can't help but feel responsible for my child's suffering."

The treatment lasted for eight months. Mansi was put on maintenance therapy after which she was to be taken for regular check-ups. Since her immunity was compromised, extreme care had to be taken to ensure that she did not catch any infections and her diet tweaked to make her strong.

Based on his experience, Manas offers the following advice for caregivers:

> ➤ "During Mansi's treatment, I was constantly thinking 'will she survive?' Such thoughts will only distract you from the important things. Don't overthink. Trust your doctor, and leave the rest in the hands of

God. Then, focus on what you need to do and never give up.

➢ The medical reports are the only indicators of the patient's health. So, give the reports more importance than the opinions of relatives and friends.

➢ Sometimes people end up saying stuff that causes you anxiety. At such times, you need to remind yourself that only if you are strong, can your loved one be strong. Take care of your body and mind.

➢ Each one has to find their own path in their journey with cancer. What worked for one, may not work for another. Hence find out what works for you and the patient. You are the best judge of that, so trust yourself. Of course, it is not easy. Cancer is no child's play.

➢ Even if it all looks too difficult and confusing right now, with time, it is possible to overcome anything. We just need to stay focussed and not give up."

9
Pursuing a Passion

The one thing that you have that nobody else has is you. Your voice, your mind, your story, your vision. So, write and draw and build and play and dance and live as only you can.
　　　　　　　　　　　　—NEIL GAIMAN, *English Author*

Pursue a passion—music, painting, gardening, reading, cooking *et al.* This will keep your mind occupied in a productive activity and will not allow negative thoughts and anxieties to invade your space.

As Barbara W. Fishman, artist and philanthropist says, "For me knowing that I was seriously ill opened doors and opportunities that have truly enriched my life. It is through cancer that I have discovered my love of painting and refocused my energies to help others. Both have given me meaningful strength and satisfaction. There is a positive side in that cancer often serves as a wake-up call that life is precious and each moment should be appreciated."

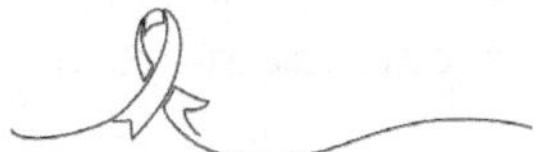

Case Study I: Suleika Jaouad, American writer, advocate, and motivational speaker

Suleika was diagnosed with a rare form of acute myeloid leukaemia in 2011. Doctors said she had only a 35 percent chance of surviving. She had to undergo a bone morrow transplant and ended up with two blood infections and excruciating combination of kidney issues and mucositis. Since she had a white blood cell count of zero, she knew she could easily die.

In her memoir *Between Two Kingdoms: A Memoir of a Life Interrupted*, Suleika writes that what saved her in those hardest moments was her passion for painting.

"When I was painting, I didn't have full awareness of what I was doing. The border between conscious and subconscious was as porous as it's ever been for me. I was taking what felt most frightening and fragile and finding a way to coexist with it. Rendering my medical situation in different landscapes and locales was a way to acknowledge my immediate reality, but also to make room for other possibilities. It only occurs to me that in these paintings, I was establishing a visual language for holding both hardship and hope in one palm.

My foray into painting continues to amaze me. Not only did it guide me through my darkest valley, it also changed me. Because of this practice, I see and engage with the world differently. I take in everything, whether the buildings on my block or the sky's particular shade of blue or the flowering trees. Rather than rushing from one thing to another, I'm slower, more purposeful. I listen, watch, and observe more intensely. I feel more curious, more alive."

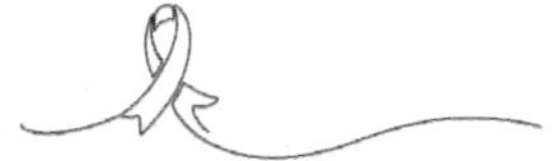

Case Study II: Ramen's experience

I have always been passionate about writing, storytelling, public speaking and dancing.

In between my radiation cycles Ankita casually mentioned that we should do a dance-video together, something crazy and cool! Seeing the unadulterated joy on my face, right there and then she conceptualised the video!

The next day, after I returned home from radiation, we got into the act. Both of us changed seven dresses and danced to the 1980s chartbuster song *'Jawaani Jaaneman, Haseen Dilruba'*. The entire 'shooting' was done in a single take. I choreographed the song, while Aniket played the cinematographer. Ankita edited the video and posted it the next day! Her Instagram post read:

"@25ramendra, my dad has just been diagnosed with second stage Cancer. He is one of the strongest, most positive, hardcore people I know. And dancing gives him the most joy, so we had to do this." The video went viral and notched up 2.25k views on Instagram in 24 hours and is still trending and at last check, the count was 234k.

In the meanwhile, Dr. Nisha, my radiation Oncologist shared the dance video, calling me a rockstar with nerves of steel and a 'humerus' which is alive and nudging:

"Ramen, a dear patient of mine, who is a celebrated author and a motivational speaker, sent me this video. I was taken aback since his world has recently been rocked upon by a cancer diagnosis and overwhelming information about treatment, side effects and uncertain outcomes. He decides to find 'humour in tumour' and sings on the radiation table, cracks jokes and makes music videos. I respect his attitude and am posting the video so that my colleagues can share with their patients as an example of how someone can dance in swag through the cancer treatment."

After I was discharged from the hospital it took me just two weeks to set up regular trysts with my writing.

I set about creating a routine for myself. I would get up late in the morning, have breakfast and then sit down to write. I would then have my lunch, watch some television, and go for my evening walk or swim. In between I would do a bit of reading and spend time on social media.

I have been conducting writing workshops, storytelling sessions, participating in panel discussions, interacting on social media with complete enthusiasm. Two months after being declared cancer free I started participating in literary festivals in different parts of the country.

I have heard numerous gurus talk of meditation as a great way of achieving mindfulness. I found my mindfulness in my passions. When I am following my Ikigai, I am completely in the moment, oblivious to the chaos within and without.

10

Moving from Fear to Faith

Fear is the mind-killer.
Fear is the little-death that brings total obliteration.
I will face my fear.
I will permit it to pass over me and through me.
And when it has gone past, I will turn the inner eye to see its path.
Where the fear has gone there will be nothing.
Only I will remain....

　　　　　　　—Frank Herbert, *American science fiction writer*

According to Manoj Sharma, author of *Introspective Meditations for Complete Contentment (Santosha)*, Yogiraj Vethathiri Maharishi, an Indian philosopher, in his approach of Simplified Kundalini Yoga (SKY) classifies fears into four categories: to be faced, to be solved immediately, to be postponed and to be ignored.

Fears to be faced include things like death, disability or other happenings that cannot be changed. Fears to be solved immediately include events like sickness for which urgent treatment is needed. Fears that need to be postponed include facets for which there is no immediacy. Finally, are the fears to be ignored that include trivial matters regarding which we have simply made it a habit to be fearful. Classifying worries or fears into such categorisation reduces the number to a manageable few and helps in facing the important ones that need to be tackled.

In an article entitled 'When facing cancer, feed your faith, not your fears,' by 'City of Hope', it is mentioned that for many people, spiritual strength is critical in the fight against cancer. It can help in maintaining a sense of hope, faith and courage while facing the ogre of cancer.

The article goes on to elaborate that a major step in getting strong spiritually is to make peace in three main areas of life. First is to make peace with yourself—you did not cause this situation so be gentle on yourself.

Next, make peace with others, spiritually. Forgive others and let go of the past. Thirdly, make peace with the Supreme Power. God did not give you cancer. Focusing on "Why, God?" will lead to frustration. Try to put that question on hold and make peace with God.

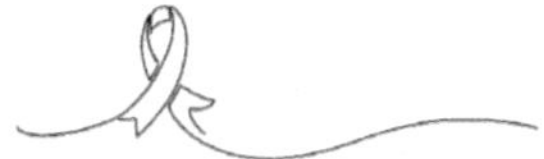

Case Study I: Sonali Bendre

Sonali Bendre, the popular Bollywood actress, announced in July 2018 that she had been diagnosed with fourth stage cancer and her chance of survival was only around 30 percent.

She tweeted: "Sometimes, when you least expect it, life throws you a curveball. I have recently been diagnosed with a high-grade cancer that has metastasised, which we frankly did not see coming. A niggling pain led to some tests, which led to this unexpected diagnosis."

Sonali expressed her gratitude to her family and friends for the outpouring of love and support. "We remain optimistic and I am determined to fight every step of the way. I'm taking this battle head-on, knowing I have the strength of my family and friends behind me."

She underwent treatment which entailed chemotherapy and surgery in New York and Mumbai. In January, much to the relief of her fans, Sonali came out with the statement that she was under remission and had returned to India.

Even while facing the toughest of odds the actress remained upbeat. She shared updates on her journey, inspiring others facing a similar crisis.

"The first thing that my doctors were telling me was that we want you out of the hospital as fast as possible. Post-surgery, my surgeon was like, I want you walking in 24 hours. In 24 hours, I was holding my IV and walking in the corridor. It was hard because I had a cut which is 23–24 inches."

According to Sonali, the specific reason why she went completely open and transparent about her battle with the deadly malady was to fight the negativity and fear around it. "I think we have to just adapt. We are in the age where information is available at our fingertips. I would just say that I didn't want any pessimism or rumours about it. Also, because my son was 12 at that point of time and kids today keep getting information from the internet, I didn't want something negative to reach him. What was happening was weird and scary enough, I didn't want to add to that. I didn't want my family members receiving some strange WhatsApp messages and getting frightened. So, the idea was to put out what is happening so that there is no speculation."

A couple of years after her recovery Sonali wrote, "How time flies...today when I look back, I see strength, I see weakness but most importantly I see the will to not let the

C word define how my life will be after it. You create the life you choose. The journey is what you make of it…so remember to take one day at a time and to switch on the sunshine."

Four years later Sonali visited the hospital in New York where she had been treated and in a poignant post shared her feelings. "This chair, this view, this exact same spot… four years later. From sheer terror to continued hope, so much has changed yet so much remains the same. It was unreal to sit there and see patients going in and I could see that I had been through a similar journey… Saw the chemotherapy suite, the same waiting room, faces were different."

In an emotional vein she added, "I felt like telling the patients that there's HOPE, and look at me today I have come in for a visit on the other side of the spectrum… It was, as you can guess, a very bittersweet, emotional day. I stepped out, looked my son in the eye, with sunshine on my face and thanked the universe for everything."

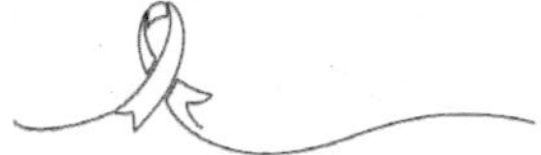

Case Study II: Ramen's experience

In November 2021, I was diagnosed with Colon Cancer. The big surgery—Colostomy—in which my colon was removed went off fine. I went home in four days, healed well so the doctors decided to go ahead with the Ileostomy reversal.

This procedure was a much, much simpler operation that turned into a complete nightmare. As one of the surgeons said, it was like surviving one accident and walking straight into another the same day.

I suffered a septic shock a week after the surgery. The doctors gave up and asked my family to visit me in the ICU.

I was lying unconscious and was on a ventilator. My palms and feet were blue and my body bloated. The BP had plummeted to 55 and wasn't picking up despite the strongest medicines known to doctors.

My daughter Ankita held my hand and started talking to me. It seemed a crazy thing to do. But in this madness the line between the rational and the irrational had blurred completely.

The scene was straight out of a Bollywood potboiler—the protagonist on the deathbed, his vitals going berserk, the others reaching out to the Almighty and waiting for the miracle to happen, which on celluloid always did. But this was not reel life, it was real life.

"Anki, it is too late for all this. He can't even hear you," my son Aniket, the most pragmatic member of my family said. He thought Ankita was losing it.

"I don't care," she replied and still holding my limp hand in hers continued.

"Papa, you are our hero. You can fight this. You have fought through so much in life, this is nothing for you. You can do it because your mind is so strong. And you have always told us that it is always the mind which rules the body. And you have to now fight with your mind.

You will fight this, Papa. You are a fighter. The strongest person I know. The person I love the MOST in my life. We all love you and we are here for you, beside you, fighting alongside you. But YOU have to fight the hardest. You've overcome so much in life. You have battled the odds and always come out a winner. And you will do the same now.

You have been so strong through this whole ordeal, Papa. We all believe in you. You have soooo much love in your life. Your family, friends, fans—people are in awe of you. You will continue to awe us with your sense of humour in adversity, your willpower and the ability to fight it all. We love you. I love you."

To their absolute amazement, my family started seeing the BP slowly go up. Soon Aniket and Madhavi also joined in, to lift my spirits. With every little milestone in the BP rise they would cheer me. For 40 minutes they spoke to me despite me being on ventilator and totally knocked out. Finally, when the BP climbed to 117, the doctors came in and took charge of the situation.

Who says miracles don't happen? When everyone had given up hope, my princess had created a connect which was sublime and surreal.

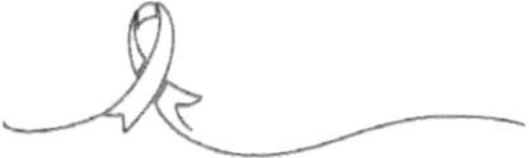

Case Study III: Gautam

Gautam, a cancer warrior, talks about how the mind-body approach to healing helped him develop resilience and battle the dreaded disease.

"Throughout my treatment, each day I would affirm the presence of the spirit and allow it to heal me. I still practice that every morning when I go out for my walk.

I look at the magnificent sun and just try to visualise that its warm and powerful rays are healing every cell in my body. I also thank the universe for giving me another beautiful day to live my life to the fullest.

While I was undergoing treatment, I had 100 percent faith in my doctor and also the medicines that were given to me. I completely believed that what my doctor is doing is the best thing for me and neither then nor now do I have any doubts or second thoughts on that.

It was a similar feeling that a child down with fever has when her father/mother touches her forehead. I felt the same way. The doctor wasn't just treating me for the disease, he was also healing me at the same time.

God touches you in many forms and my doctor was just one of the instruments sent by God. Since my chemo cycles were spaced between a gap of three weeks, strangely enough I would just look forward to visiting the hospital and getting the next cycle done.

The universe surely has mysterious ways of working. In order to receive the gifts from the universe we just need to believe and it starts at the cellular level.

The moment you start believing that I'm in safe hands and the universe is taking care of me, that micro-step is the stepping stone to a major life transforming change. The energy that one experiences is phenomenal.

What you choose to believe is directly correlated to the amount of magic you experience in your life."

11

Taking Humour, Seriously

If you laugh at misfortune, you will not be overcome by it.
                        —VALLUVAR, *Tamil poet–sage*

Jennifer Aaker and Naomi Bagdonas in their book *Humour, Seriously* say, "A sense of humour is part of what makes us human. It's a deeply connecting and empowering thing. Deploying it doesn't make light of serious things. It means you're able to move forward, in spite of those serious things."

In a research article titled 'The impact of humour on patients with cancer' published in *National Library of Medicine*, Wanda Christie and Carole Moore write that using the Stetler model, in-depth literature reviews were performed that demonstrated a positive correlation between humour and comfort levels in patients with cancer. Humour frequently was used for relaxation and as a coping mechanism that aided in promoting general wellness. The literature indicated that various types of humorous material lessened anxiety and discomfort, which allowed for patients' concerns and fears to be discussed openly. The literature also showed that humour had a positive effect on the immune system. Improvements in pain thresholds and elevations in natural killer cell activity (Killer T cells are types of white blood cells which are separated from other blood cells, grown in the laboratory and then given to a patient to kill cancer cells) consistently appeared in experimental studies. In addition, research also revealed improved response to stress and increased feelings of well-being after humorous interventions.

According to Saranne Rothberg who founded The ComedyCures Foundation from her chemo chair in 1999 and is still cancer-free, "Research shows that finding the funny in one's cancer journey and developing a comic perspective are powerful stress management coping strategies."

Here it would be pertinent to talk about a movie which is a must watch for every individual who believes in the dignity of humour.

Life is Beautiful is a cinematic experience I would cherish for a long time to come. In it the protagonist is deported to Auschwitz, the dreaded Nazi concentration camp along with his seven-year-old son. There, instead of wallowing in pity or cursing fate, the father uses all his creativity and ingenuity in making 'life beautiful' for his young son.

Rather than turning out to be an ordeal the experience becomes fun for the child thanks to the guts, gumption and inventiveness of the father. Ultimately the father dies and, in the process, teaches the son (and the viewers) the value of life and living.

The film is a classic example of how humour can be used in the most horrendous of circumstances to heal, educate and elevate. We can and we should indulge in humour to deal with the 'concentration camps' in our day-to-day life to emerge unscathed.

In the article 'Keeping your sense of humour during cancer treatment', Edward-Elmhurst Health points out that laughter has always been the best medicine, but maintaining a sense of humour can be a real challenge when you're going through cancer treatment.

"It's not always easy dealing with the different emotions that come with cancer and its treatment. Working through your feelings—and finding ways to laugh a little—can help reduce your stress level and improve your mental health. Cancer is no laughing matter, but humour therapy can help you feel better by making you less stressed, worried or anxious."

The writer suggests the following elements of humour therapy which can bring more laughter into the life of a cancer patient:

> Find something you enjoy doing that makes you laugh—watch funny movies or videos, look at funny photos, read comic strips or jokes, or take part in your favourite fun activity.

> Practice positivity by challenging the negative thoughts in your mind. Try writing down three things you are thankful for each day.

> Find a way to manage your stress such as Yoga. Spend time with a funny friend. You can also find strength by sharing your thoughts and feelings in a support group with others who are going through a similar experience.

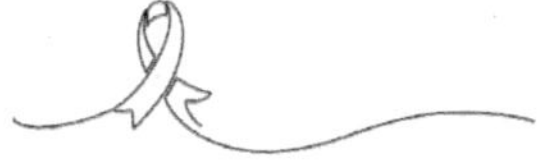

Case Study I: Ramen's experience

Throughout the treatment I shared my journey with my offline and online friends with my trademark humour. While the response of most of them was positive, there was a flip side to my sharing as well.

A 'well-wisher', a doctor, advised me just as I was getting ready for my first major surgery, "Ramen, while so far you have been sharing your experience with everyone, it is now a time to do a serious rethink. After your operation you have to start looking inwards, this will help you energise your cells."

I laughed and replied, "Bro, for the last six months I feel half of the city has been peering into my rectum and I feel that it has got almost as many eyeballs as the *Natu-Natu* song. How much more inwards should I look?"

But the crumb, the cake and the casserole go to an aged relative of mine who told Madhavi, "Has Ramen gone mad? Why is he indulging in all this nonsense on social media? He is making a mockery of cancer. Does he not know death is no laughing matter? If he continues, he will die in bits and pieces."

I told Madhavi, "Please reply to him that I will not allow the lack of a colon to put a period, a comma or even a semi-colon to my humour and creativity!

Also, that 2022 seems to be the year of the comedian—Zelenskyy in Ukraine, Bhagwant Mann in Punjab and hopefully Ramendra Kumar in Bangalore. And, finally, convey to him that I believe in two great philosophers—Gabbar who said in 1975, '*Jo darr gaya samjho mar gaya*' and Pushpa in 2022 who declared '*Main jhukega nahin*'."

I was also 'accused' by another very erudite friend of practising the 'tyranny of cheerfulness'.

I have realised that there will always be individuals who will question or castigate my response to cancer. But rather than getting mired in their opinion and feeling demoralised I have decided to shrug the negativity, embrace my credo and unleash as much joy as I possibly can.

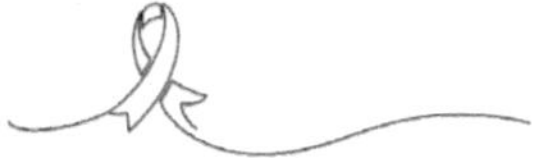

Case Study II: Pallavi Aiyar

Pallavi, a journalist and author, is a breast cancer survivor.

When Pallavi was diagnosed with breast cancer she never allowed it to overwhelm her. Like the protagonist of *Life is Beautiful,* she created a world of humour, gentle wisdom and resilience for her kids.

While undergoing treatment she wrote in her newsletter *The Global Jigsaw*, "How does one say farewell to a part of oneself? In my case, this is quite literal as I will have a radical mastectomy later this afternoon. It's been a good breast, tingling pleasurably at the appropriate moments, and feeding my babes when needed. So, I bid it goodbye with sadness, but also the knowledge that impermanence is the way of the world; and that appreciation is deepened by finiteness.

My breast goes the way of cherry blossoms in Japan. *Sakura* (Japanese for Cherry Blossom Trees) evoke *mono no aware* (Japanese idiom for the awareness of impermanence) which, roughly speaking, is the pain we feel at the end of something beautiful, mixed up with knowledge that transience is an essential part of their beauty. Mine is not the world's most beautiful mammary, but today it will be gorgeous, in the very moment it is scooped and cut and discarded."

The day Pallavi learnt she had breast cancer she was on a vacation with her family, on an island off the coast of northern Spain.

The news came in the form of a phone call, informing her that a mammogram she'd had a few days earlier, showed a highly suspicious mass requiring an immediate biopsy. Over the next two months she went to the hospital more than 30 times, had two biopsies, a lumpectomy and was now scheduled for further surgery and months of chemotherapy. In three, short-long months, she had transformed from the mother who pulls her children up mountains and laughs into the wind, into the mother who has to excuse herself from dinner at restaurants, to have a cry in the loo.

She goes on to write, "What is the proper comportment to adopt when breaking the news of serious illness to one's children? You want to collapse with grief at the loss of your health, but you also want to protect your beautiful boys with all your fierce might. You want to reassure them that everything will be ok, despite the niggling knowledge that it might not be. And you want them to reassure you that everything will be ok, even though how could they know? It's a mess of emotions to calibrate."

Pallavi and her husband mostly adopted a matter-of-fact tone while discussing her illness: "Mama is not going to die. It will be tough, but we'll pull together, and she will get better."

When her kids witnessed her distraught, heaving with volcanic hurt, she would tell them it was a process. They should all allow themselves to feel the sad feelings, so they can settle into something akin to determination. She might cry sometimes, but she also laughs and sings and takes pleasure in life and books and words and autumn and them.

She narrates the response of her two boys. "My 14-year-old has researched the histology of my particular carcinoma and is convinced of an excellent prognosis. He sneaks up on me and gives me giant hugs, even though he's not big on physical affection. He balances the out-of-character niceness by cackling as he informs me that I'm soon going to look like a bald, boob-less man (which I am not, thanks to breast reconstruction and my general feminine elegance).

My 11-year-old makes me steaming cups of green tea and gives me foot massages, which I (lightly) exploit my cancer to extract from him in plentiful measure.

My husband has the boys helping with cooking dinner, cleaning up and feeding the cats. There are times they don't like the extra chores. When they complain, it takes a slightly tragic look from me, for them to become contrite, at least for the few minutes it takes to clear the table."

Talking about facing chaos and thriving on it Pallavi says, "A crisis is a time of assessment. And much as it is about pain and fear, it can also be a time of an abundance of love, a richness of kindness, and a renewed determination to focus on the wonderful things. It has forged of my family a unit. One that quibbles and whines and has off days, but that together, is more than the sum of its parts.

No one would want to have cancer or wish it on anyone else. But what I do wish is for us to not waste the challenge in self-pity and anxiety over outcomes we can't control. I want my family and me to learn resilience, gratitude for the good stuff and acceptance of the bad shit. I want my boys to understand the importance of caring for their own health and to nurture the skills of empathy and nursing that boys, in particular, often lack.

We are all travelling into new terrain. It's not the most hospitable of places perhaps, but every new place has something to teach us, if only we have the eyes to look and learn."

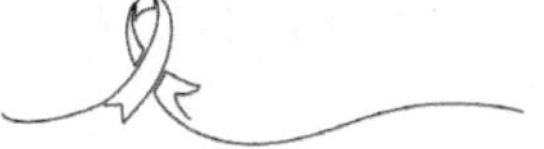

12

A Tribute

I would like to conclude with my tribute to all cancer patients and their caregivers who prove what I have always believed in: "The worst of times often bring out the best in us."

THE CANCER WARRIORS

As I stumbled through the dark night
With not a shard in sight,
The black became blacker
The night a darker night.

I had plunged into despair
From a state of happiest high,
Fighting a malady that was
Smothering my every sigh.

'Why me?' 'Poor me'
I raved and ranted,
Then I saw three anxious faces
The look in their eyes so haunted.

I decided to fight the scourge
Slam the damn tumour,
With my precious weapons
Of masti and humour.

My three hearts ensnared me
In a web of optimism and love,
It was as if three amazing angels
Had descended from heavens above.

Now sheathed in their empathy
And cloaked in their affection,
I can fight any malady
Battle the worst affliction.

Tons of heart-warming messages
From friends, followers and 'fans',
Have been like myriad oases
In arid, desert sands.

These zillion tiny rainbows
Have caressed my soul,
Helping me march
Towards my only goal.

No cancer can beat me
No malady can crush,
When I have the invincible army
Of You, Me and Us!

I am not a cancer 'survivor'
You are not a cancer saviour,
Each one of us is
Simply a Cancer Warrior!

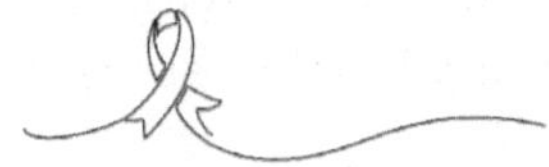

13

FAQs

1. **How can the cancer patients and their caregivers manage their finances while they go in for the best treatment?**

   Cancer is slowly and surely becoming a pandemic. The treatment is often long, arduous and puts a severe strain on the finances. Everyone needs to have an insurance cover/ savings so that he/she can manage the huge financial crisis which he/she is bound to face post the diagnosis, treatment and recovery.

2. **What are the health protocols that need to be followed during treatment and after recovery?**

   It is extremely important to stringently follow the schedule of visits to the hospital, diet, exercise regimen *et al* prescribed by the doctors. There is no scope for any laxity whatsoever.

   'Coping Strategies' suggested in the book can be of immense help to cancer patients/care givers during the treatment as well as post recovery.

3. **Are there any particular traits which can make coping with cancer easier?**

   According to Jimmie C. Holland MD, research has shown that the following qualities can help a person cope better:

   - A positive attitude
   - Ability to take one day at a time

> Capability to meet any challenge head-on
> Attitude to see the humorous side of negative things
> Having a personal belief that gives a holistic perspective in tough situations.

4. **What are the Organisations/NGOs/Support Groups in the field of cancer awareness and care?**

> Indian Cancer Society: https://www.indiancancersociety.org/
> My Healing Mate: https://www.myhealingmate.com/resources
> ONCO: https://onco.com/
> PatientsEngage: https://www.patientsengage.com/
> YouWeCan: https://youwecan.org/
> Tanisa Foundation: https://www.tanisafoundation.org/
> Sanjeevani: https://www.sanjeevani-lifebeyondcancer.com/
> https://www.cancerassist.in/support-groups-for-cancer-patients
> CanSupport: https://cansupport.org/
> SoulUp: https://www.soulup.in/

References

1. Susan Sontag, *Illness As Metaphor*, Penguin Modern Classics, 2009.

2. Ramendra Kumar & Dr. Sandeep Nayak, 'Triumph Over Rectal Cancer: A Journey of Resilience, https://www.youtube.com/watch?v=fArgL7sTt9g

3. Ramendra Kumar, 'Creating an Ecosystem of Positivity after Cancer Diagnosis', https://copingmag.com/creating-an-ecosystem-of-positivity-after-a-cancer-diagnosis/

4. Manoj Sharma, *Introspective Meditations for Complete Contentment (Santosha)*, Published by Health for All, Inc, Omaha, Nebraska

5. Lachlan Brown, 'The art of not caring: 8 simple ways to live a happy life', https://geediting.com/the-art-of-not-caring-8-simple-ways-to-live-a-happy-life-2/

6. 'Together Against Cancer: Mukta, a Cancer Caregiver, Shares Her Story', https://onco.com/blog/together-against-cancer-mukta-a-cancer-caregiver-shares-her-story/

7. Pallavi Aiyar, Switching passports to the kingdom of the sick, *Voices, Lifestyle, TOI*, October 3, 2022, https://timesofindia.indiatimes.com/blogs/voices/switching-passports-to-the-kingdom-of-the-sick/?source=app&frmapp=yes

8. Francesc Miralles and Héctor García, *The Book of Ichigo Ichie*, Quercus, 2020

9. Lillian Eichler Watson, *Light From Many Lamps*, Simon & Schuster, January 1988

10. Jimmie C. Holland MD and Sheldon Lewis, The Human Side of Cancer by, Harper Perennial, 2001

11. 'Sutras/Discourse on Knowing the Better Way to Live Alone', https://plumvillage.org/library/sutras/discourse-on-knowing-the-better-way-to-live-alone

12. Surabhi Kakkar, 'My Brush with Cancer', *There is Life After Cancer*, Jyotsna Govil (ed.), Vitasta and Indian Cancer Society, Delhi

13. Jessica Reid Sliwerski, 'What cancer taught me about living in the moment', https://www.headspace.com/articles/embracing-cancer-a-new-mom-finds-strength-in-the-present

14. Fereshteh Ahmadi, Mohammad Khodayarifard, Mohammad Rabbani, *et al.*, Existential Meaning-Making Coping in Iran: A Qualitative Study among Patients with Cancer, February 22, 2022, https://www.mdpi.com/2076-0760/11/2/80

15. NDTV, 'Sanjay Dutt Reveals He Initially Did Not Want Treatment After Cancer Diagnosis,' https://www.ndtv.com/entertainment/i-don-t-want-any-treatment-sanjay-dutt-shares-his-first-reaction-to-cancer-diagnosis-3689142

16. Rinku Ghosh, 'How Sanjay Dutt defeated cancer with precision treatment, will power and not getting off the treadmill even on chemo days', February 8, 2023, https://indianexpress.com/article/health-wellness/world-cancer-day-how-sanjay-dutt-defeated-cancer-with-precision-treatment-will-power-and-not-getting-off-the-treadmill-even-on-chemo-days-8423376/

17. Neerja Chowdhury, 'Just a Hiccup in the journey of life', *There is Life After Cancer*, Jyotsna Govil (ed.), Vitasta and Indian Cancer Society, Delhi.

18. Ramendra Kumar, 'Managing My Siamese Twin (Stoma Bag), https://www.patientsengage.com/personal-voices/managing-my-stoma-bag-colon-cancer

19. Martin Seligman, Martin Seligman & Positive Psychology, https://www.pursuit-of-happiness.org/history-of-happiness/martin-seligman-psychology/

20. Dr. Vijay Anand Reddy, *I am a Survivor, 108 stories of Triumph Over Cancer*, Penguin, 2017.

21. *Economic Times*, 'Cancer taught Manisha Koirala to value life; actress said disease made her kinder, gentler', https://economictimes.indiatimes.com/magazines/panache/cancer-taught-manisha-koirala-to-value-life-actress-said-disease-made-her-kinder-gentler/articleshow/67721183.cmsutm_source=contentofinterest&utm_medium=text&utm_campaign=cppst

22. Suhani Singh, 'There is no bitterness to my cancer experience,' says Manisha Koirala, https://www.indiatoday.in/movies/bollywood/story/manisha-koirala-talks-about-cancer-experience-life-and-bollywood-films-179203-2014-01-31

23. *Hindustan Times*, 'Manisha Koirala writes about 'arduous' fight with cancer, shares pics from her treatment', https://www.hindustantimes.com/entertainment/bollywood/manisha-koirala-writes-about-arduous-fight-with-cancer-shares-pics-from-her-treatment-101636291740339.html

24. https://www.tanisafoundation.org/

25. Anshul Chaturvedi, Irrfan Khan on battling cancer: 'I trust, I've surrendered, Irrespective of the outcome', TNN, June 9, 2018, https://timesofindia.indiatimes.com/entertainment/hindi/bollywood/news/irrfan-on-battling-cancer-i-trust-ive-surrendered-irrespective-of-the-outcome/articleshow/64635045.cms?from=mdr

26. Neena Singh, 'The Second Chance', *There is Life After Cancer*, Jyotsna Govil (ed.), Vitasta and Indian Cancer Society, Delhi

27. Marylin French, *A Season In Hell*, Open Royal Media, 2018

28. Dr. Rashmi HR, *Holistic Happy You: 15 Powerful Daily Habits That Transform Your Life To Healthy & Happy You*, Notion Press, 2022

29. Ramendra Kumar, Papa's Day Out: How He Built Lifetime Memories With His Kids, Kidsstoppress, September 8, 2023, https://kidsstoppress.com/dad-memories-stories-kids/

30. Nasrin Modak Siddiqi, "This cancer survivor who lost her mom shares a key life lesson on grief and joy", July 23, 2023, https://www.mid-day.com/sunday-mid-day/article/love-loss-and-a-jar-of-joy-23299455

31. Daniel Goleman, *Emotional Intelligence*, Bloomsbury Publishing India Private Limited, 1995

32. Brigadier S.C. Sharma, 'The Fourth War', *There is Life After Cancer*, Jyotsna Govil (ed.), Vitasta and Indian Cancer Society, Delhi

33. Asha Choudhry, 'Beginning a New Life', *There is Life After Cancer*, Jyotsna Govil (ed.), Vitasta and Indian Cancer Society, Delhi

34. Venkat Rao Pulla, Kiran Kumar Keshavamurthy Salagame, 'Wellbeing: Through the Lens of Indian Traditional Conceptualisations', *International Journal of Social Work and Human Services Practice*, July 1, 2018, https://www.researchgate.net/publication/340921236_Wellbeing_Through_the_Lens_of_Indian_Traditional_Conceptualisations

35. Scroll, Down but not out: Yuvraj Singh's comeback from cancer—the story of an indomitable spirit, April 27, 2020, https://scroll.in/field/960323/against-all-odds-yuvraj-singh-s-comeback-from-cancer-the-story-of-an-indomitable-spirit

36. ANI, 'You HAVE TO Win This Battle—Cricketer and Cancer Survivor Yuvraj Singh's heartfelt message to Cancer patients on World Cancer Day', February 04, 2022, https://www.business-standard.com/content/press-releases-ani/you-have-to-win-this-battle-cricketer-and-cancer-survivor-yuvraj-singh-s-heartfelt-message-to-cancer-patients-on-world-cancer-day-122020401080_1.html

37. Dr. Sudesh Mukhopadyaya, 'Breast Cancer Inspired Me to Live My Life', https://myemotionalhealthin.com/2019/01/11/breast-cancer-inspired-me-to-live-my-life-dr-sudesh-mukhopadyaya/

38. 'Caregiver Speak: Cancer is No Child's Play', February 26, 2020, https://onco.com/blog/caregiver-speak-cancer-is-no-childs-play/

39. Suleika Jaouad, *Between Two Kingdoms: A Memoir of a Life Interrupted*, Random House, 2021 Ramendra Kumar, 'Resilience was the only option for dealing with Colon Cancer', https://www.patientsengage.com/personal-voices/resilience-was-only-option-dealing-colon-cancer

40. City of Hope, 'When facing cancer, feed your faith, not your fears', October 13, 2015, https://www.cancercenter.com/community/blog/2015/10/feeding-your-faith

41. Manisha Chauhan, 'Didn't let the C-word define my life': When Sonali Bendre opened up about her battle with cancer', DNA, February 17, 2024, https://www.dnaindia.com/bollywood/report-didn-t-let-the-c-word-define-my-life-when-sonali-bendre-opened-up-about-her-battle-with-cancer-3078372

42. Pranita Chaubey, 'Cancer Survivor Sonali Bendre Visits The Hospital Where She Was Treated. Read Her "Bittersweet" Post', NDTV, July 13, 2022, https://www.ndtv.com/entertainment/cancer-survivor-sonali-bendre-visits-the-hospital-where-she-was-treated-read-her-bittersweet-post-3153401

43. Hindustan Times, 'Sonali Bendre says she was left with 24 inch scar post cancer surgery in 2018: 'It was hard', May 25, 2022, https://www.hindustantimes.com/entertainment/bollywood/sonali-bendre-says-she-was-left-with-24-inch-scar-post-cancer-surgery-in-2018-it-was-hard-101653465702079.html

44. Ramendra Kumar, 'Positivity and Relationships Make Each Day Worth Living', https://www.patientsengage.com/personal-voices/positivity-relationships-make-each-day-worth-living

45. Jennifer Aaker and Naomi Bagdonas, *Humour, Seriously: Why Humour Is A Superpower At Work And In Life*, Currency, 2021

46. Christie W, Moore C., The impact of humor on patients with cancer, *Clin J Oncol Nurs.* 2005 Apr;9(2):211-8. doi: 10.1188/05.CJON.211-218

47. Edward-Elmhurst Health, 'Keeping your sense of humour during cancer treatment', March 06, 2019,https://www.eehealth.org/blog/2019/03/keeping-your-sense-of-humor/#

48. Pallavi Aiyar, 'Farewell, good breast: Sakura and mammaries and talking to the children about my diagnosis', *The Global Jigsaw*, October 26, 2022, https://pallaviaiyar.substack.com/p/farewell-good-breast

About the Author

Ramendra Kumar (Ramen) is an award-winning writer, Performance Storyteller, and Inspirational Speaker with 49 books to his credit. He has written across all genres ranging from picture books to adult fiction, satire, poetry, travelogues, biographies, ghazals and on issues related to parenting and relationships. His writings have been translated into 32 languages, and have been published by major publishing houses of the country. His books brought out by National Book Trust (NBT), India, have notched up sales of more than 4.9 lakh copies in just one year.

He has participated in several international literary festivals as well as Indian events including the prestigious Jaipur Litfest.

Ramen is a cancer warrior who was diagnosed in November 2021. He survived 3 septic shocks, underwent 4 major surgeries, several rounds of chemo and radiation and was in the ICU for 40 days. He was declared 'Cancer free' in November 2022. His incredibly brave fight with this malady has become a source of inspiration to many. Throughout his treatment and post recovery, Ramen was invited to several online and offline platforms to share his amazing journey. These include Indian Cancer Society (ICS), Indian Institute of Science (IISC), Mumbai Storytellers Society, Hyderabad Literary Festival, Chennai Storytelling Festival et al.

His battle with the deadly scourge has been showcased by the hugely popular 'Humans of Bombay' and has garnered more than 4 million views. His articles, interviews and motivational videos have been published in both international and national journals as well as healthcare platforms.

An alumnus of the prestigious Hyderabad Public School (HPS), Begumpet, Ramen is an Engineer and an MBA. He was General Manager (Corporate Communications), SAIL when he took Voluntary Retirement to pursue his passion.

He can be reached on 25ramendra@gmail.com. Ramen also has a page devoted to him on Wikipedia.

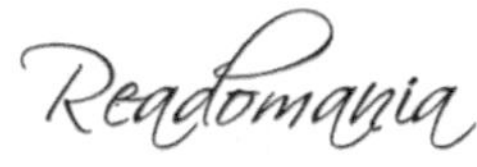

Readomania exists to nurture, curate, and bring to you content you love. We are a publishing house that takes pride in encouraging talent, new or old, and provide a wonderful platform for awesome stories.

We make this possible in multiple ways.

The first as an independent publishing house. Readomania boasts of multiple imprints across various categories—fiction, nonfiction, children, to name a few. An eclectic mix of content for its readers, when you read a Readomania title, you enter a world that's yours, supported by unique and quality narratives.

The second, as an online publishing platform for writers—a place to share stories, poems, opinions, travelogues, a way to explore your creative talent. Available as premium, as well as free-to-read content across multiple genres, the reader is spoilt for choice.

Join us in this journey, as we explore, develop, and present stories to our readers and audiences. Welcome to the world of Readomania, get ready to craft stories that enrich lives.

You can visit us at: www.readomania.com